The Girlfriend's Guide to Lupus

The Girlfriend's Guide to Lupus

How to Control Your Shitty Diagnosis

Amanda Chay

The Girlfriend's Guide to Lupus:

How to Control Your Shitty Diagnosis

ISBN: 9798861226141

Cover and illustrations design by Khanh Du Nguyen

Author photo by Rishelle Barber

Dedication

For my daughter, Ahnna,

who has lupus and is totally badass.

Contents

To create one's own world
takes courage.

—Georgia O'Keeffe

Introduction

You can't give your life more days, but you can give your days more life.

—Anonymous

"Yes, you have lupus," the rheumatologist said in a deadpan voice because, you know, showing a teensy bit of empathy at a time like this would be totally out of the question. It was 2021, and there I was, nervously sitting in a rheumatology practice in Raleigh, North Carolina.

I had waited a long time for a diagnosis, and this was all the information I received. A halfway decent doctor would have taken a moment to explain what this meant for me or at least allowed me to catch my breath after delivering such devastating news before handing me a prescription for Plaquenil (the gold standard medication for lupus) and ushering me out the door.

Receiving a lupus diagnosis was both a relief and a punch in the gut. Deep down, I had known for almost a decade that something was seriously wrong with me, ever since I received my first autoimmune diagnosis. This confirmation was both validating and crushing as I mentally screamed, "Oh shit, I actually have lupus!"

I stumbled out of the medical office in a daze. "What the hell?" I thought. "Seriously, is this all I get?" A diagnosis of a chronic autoimmune disease that took ages to figure out, and all the doctor gave me was a prescription? Not even a crappy *Yippee, I Have Lupus!* bumper sticker or a boring brochure to help me navigate this freakin' nightmare?

I was confused, afraid, and alone.

And my family, oh my, they meant well. My husband, bless his hunky heart, gave me one of those "we'll get through this together" speeches that was supposed to cheer me up.

But it didn't.

I knew absolutely no one with lupus, and I was in an all-around dark place.

To make matters worse, five months after my diagnosis, my oldest daughter, Ahnna, also received a lupus diagnosis at the tender age of twenty-one. I was filled with anxiety and worry, and I blamed myself for her illness. I felt like I was drowning in a sea of mom guilt.

Carl Jung, a famed psychiatrist, once said, "The things that worry us the most are the things we don't understand." Well, Carl, you hit the nail on the head! After months of wallowing in despair after my diagnosis, I had an epiphany: I had to come to terms with the fact that my lupus was here to stay. It was a wake-up call that propelled me into action.

I rolled up my sleeves and got to work. For me, that meant diving headfirst into research. I devoured books, medical journals, and clinical trials like candy, desperately seeking a glimpse of what my future might hold. But the reality laid out in front of me was far from pretty it was downright bleak. However, it became my mission to take control of my health and become the fiercest, most badass advocate for lupus that I could be.

I come by it naturally, it seems, as I developed a hardcore, slightly neurotic dedication to health and fitness early on, always pushing myself to be better and make the most of what my body can do. My professional career has revolved around the healthcare industry, where I trained and directed individuals and teams on aspects of medical care. I knew the value of addressing mental health and emotional concerns head on thanks to my master's degree in counseling. And for the past five years, I have owned a stress reduction and mindfulness business, helping countless companies better manage stress.

After overcoming the initial shock of my diagnosis, I felt a deep sense of gratitude toward the lupus community that generously supported me as I made my way through those first frightening months and years after my diagnosis. It was clear that I had to give back in any way I could. I've had the opportunity to stand on Capitol Hill, speak to members of

Congress, and advocate for the rights of those with lupus. I've also dedicated my time as a volunteer on statewide executive lupus teams and served as a shareholder on a university lupus board.

The inspiration for *The Girlfriend's Guide to Lupus* came from the idea that the same knowledge and tools I had used to take care of my own autoimmune diseases could be combined with what I'd learned about lupus to help other women who were going through the same struggles.

During the book research phase, I dug deep into the latest information on lupus, autoimmune diseases, nutrition, sleep, and exercise that would guide me on this quest. I compiled resources and conducted interviews with esteemed professionals, including rheumatologists, scientists, physical therapists, and nutritionists. Also, I made a point to connect with women who graciously shared their own experiences, both the highs and lows.

Consider me one of those believers who finds purpose in life's twists and turns. I've waited, pondered, hoped, and prayed for a reason why this shitty lupus has come along. It is clear to me now: I am here to stand beside you, to shine a little bit of light and hope so that you can find your own way with lupus.

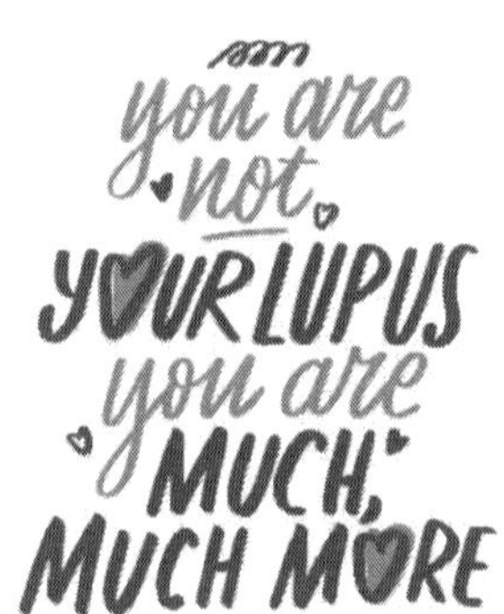

In this book, I'll share all the knowledge, experience, and tips that I wish someone had shared with me when I was diagnosed. **The more you understand yourself and how lupus shows up for you, the better you'll be able to manage it and elevate parts of your health.**

This book is in your hands, my reader friend, to ease some worry on your quest and help you take control of a shitty diagnosis. To guide you toward finding your deepest health by making the best decisions for you. To empower you to live a life that is not limited by lupus but alive with lupus. Because there is a difference, and you deserve all of this and more. Everything your big, amazing heart desires.

With *The Girlfriend's Guide to Lupus*, you will learn:

- how to be a badass and stand up for your medical needs (Chapter 4)
- why your daily habits totally make up your health (Chapter 7)
- how sex changes after diagnosis (Chapter 14)
- how staying in the present is so much better for you and your lupus (Chapter 17)
- what foods to devour and which to cross off your list (Chapter 19)

And so much freakin' more.

Take What You Need

Even though this book is based on what has helped me deal with my lupus, you can take as much or as little from it as you want. Know that I am not an expert who can tell you how to make your lupus go away. In fact, no one can do this. I am here to spill the beans on what has helped me stay healthy and happy. If it helps you, that is great. If something strikes a chord, investigate it further. Leave anything that is not right for you behind.

If you are looking for an intensive clinical dive into lupus, then this isn't the best book for you. May I recommend Donald Thomas, Jr., M.D.'s 874-page book, *The Lupus Encyclopedia*. It can boost your medical knowledge and kill a cockroach with its weight alone. Check out the book recommendation section at the back of the book for more information.

Caregivers and Support Team

If someone you care about has lupus and you're reading this, kudos to you. Way to support your loved one! This book will help you better understand what that person is going through. Your importance in her life cannot be overstated—you can be a lifeline during dark times. Your presence alone provides a sense of stability and enhances the quality of life for your loved one with lupus. Simply put, you rock!

Disclaimer

The Girlfriend's Guide to Lupus is not designed to replace any rheumatological and/or medical care. Your physicians know best. Trust them with your lupus medical care. Don't stop (or start) any medications or therapies without their knowledge. The goal of this book is to deepen your understanding of lupus and what parts of your health you can control through education, awareness, and inspiration. Now let's get on with this thing.

1

Lupus: She's a Maniacal Meanie!

Lupus is one of the cruelest, most mysterious diseases—an unpredictable and misunderstood autoimmune disease that ravages different parts of the body... It is difficult to diagnose, hard to live with, a challenge to treat, and can be fatal.

—Lupus Foundation of America

My lupus symptoms unofficially started during a very challenging pregnancy with my first daughter, which involved seven hospitalizations, multiple feeding tubes, and serious drug allergies. At one point, my obstetrician said my life would be at risk if my body couldn't get its act together.

I survived the pregnancy and gave birth to a healthy baby girl, Ahnna. A few years later, my knees began to ache. I ignored this pain and blamed it on all the years I'd spent running around on soccer fields and tracks. Ulcers began to show up in my mouth, but my dentist shrugged and said it was probably normal. I took her lack of concern as a good thing and pressed on.

Time passed, and I had another sweet daughter named Kaia, this time without as many issues. As my girls grew up, pulsating pain in my knees and hips became the norm. Again, naively, I thought it was my intense fitness regime to blame, or perhaps my nutrition needed a boost. I blamed myself for treating my body so poorly, even as I tried to act as though nothing were wrong.

After a move to North Carolina and a myriad of painful new symptoms, I finally went to get help. The doctor didn't find anything, but a blood panel was ordered, and I became the (un)lucky winner of my first autoimmune disease, called Sjögren's (pronounced show-grens). This is where the body often attacks the cells in the eyes and mouth, among other things, causing dryness and pain. I went to a rheumatologist for confirmation and promptly refused medication. I was strong as an ox, tough as nails, and wouldn't show any weakness. Not yet, at least. That, however, is only my story; in this book, we will pay close attention to you, your symptoms, and your path through a lupus diagnosis.

Get ready to dive into the world of lupus in this chapter. You will see how it's a confusing disease that puzzles both doctors and people who have it. Find out how this disease rears its ugly head and how hard it can be to diagnose. Prepare to swim through the murky waters of lupus, where clarity is not a given but rather earned.

Lupus Stats

Lupus is a challenging autoimmune disease. Not only can it affect any part of the body, but it's complicated, hard to diagnose, and incurable. The symptoms are all over the place, and it can be a real pain in the ass, to say the least. It's like trying to solve a Rubik's Cube blindfolded while riding a unicycle—not exactly a walk in the park, if you know what I mean. Lupus is still not well understood, and those who live with it have a lot to deal with on a multitude of levels.

Here are some statistics on lupus that are not meant to scare you, but they just may:

- 5 million people worldwide have lupus. (This number could be much higher, as it is heavily underdiagnosed.)
- 1.5 million Americans have lupus—that's a measly .45 percent of the population.
- It takes on average 5–7 years to receive a diagnosis after the first symptom arises.
- 25 to 50 percent of people suffering from lupus have more than one autoimmune disease.[1]
- It is still unknown exactly what causes lupus or how to cure it.

- Lupus is not transmissible, so you cannot give it to your annoying little sister. Aw, shucks.
- Lupus is more common in women than in men, regardless of age or ethnicity. In fact, 90 percent of all people with lupus are women, and it most often strikes between the ages of 15 and 44.

Broken Autoimmune System

Lupus is an autoimmune disease, which means your immune system gets all kinds of confused and starts attacking healthy tissues and organs. It's like that one drunk friend of yours who can't handle her alcohol, who starts fighting for no reason, and ends up wrecking the entire party. This is majorly sucky because your immune system has the important job of protecting the body and uses inflammation as a way to do this.

When your immune system is activated, it sends out inflammatory cells to attack foreign invaders or heal from damage. Let's say you cut your finger with a knife. Inflammation occurs in and around that cut as white blood cells rush in to fight off any foreign invaders. These white blood cells help you heal, and then they go to rest up for the next battle. This is how inflammation is supposed to work in a healthy system. Inflammation goes away when the body is healed or the threat is removed.

But when you have lupus, you have widespread, constant inflammation because your body continues to send out inflammatory cells despite not being sick or injured. This, in turn, wreaks all kinds of havoc on your body. When bad things (aka bacteria or viruses) do come along, your body is so exhausted from the constant battles it's fighting that some bad cells slip right into it. This is the reason why people with weakened immune systems get sick easier, stay sick longer, and are at an increased risk of serious diseases like cancer.

Lifelong Lupus

Lupus is a chronic autoimmune disease, which means it lasts a very long time, if not forever. **The reality is that lupus is here to stay with you for the duration of your life, at least until a cure is found.**

While, for the time being, you can't rid yourself of lupus, you can expect your disease activity to wax and wane, with highs and lows, kinda like Bitcoin's value. When lupus symptoms increase and the disease activity is high, this is considered a "flare." Some people flare once or twice a year, and others flare more often. When both symptoms and disease activity are absent for a set period, a person is considered to be in remission, although there's no widely agreed upon definition of remission. A person can move from remission back into lupus over and over.

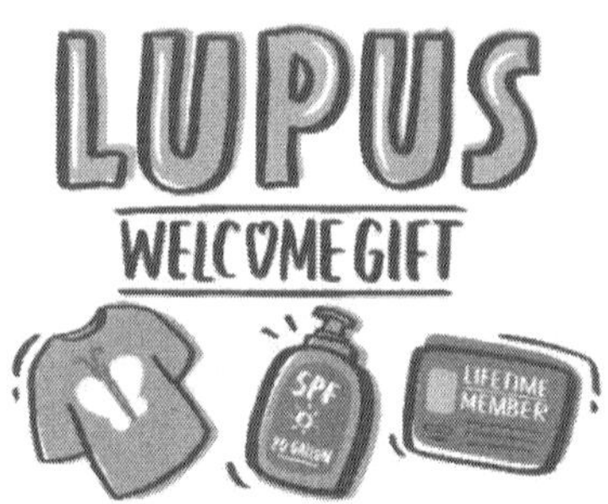

Types of Lupus

Let's talk about the different types of lupus, as there are four ways this disease rears its ugly head:

1. **Systemic lupus erythematosus* (SLE)** is the most common and serious type of lupus, accounting for 70 percent of all cases worldwide.[2] The heart, lungs, kidneys, and brain are involved in 50 percent of cases, per the Lupus Foundation of America. One of the most severe kidney complications, lupus nephritis, affects up to 50 percent of people with SLE.[3]
2. **Cutaneous lupus** affects only the skin and accounts for 10 percent of the lupus population. It typically shows up as a thick, scaly rash on the skin, face, scalp, or other parts of the body. The rash can last anywhere from a few days to several weeks and may cause scarring. The most common person with cutaneous lupus is a woman in her forties or fifties.
3. **Drug induced lupus** occurs when certain medications are taken in high doses. The symptoms experienced are similar to those of SLE but return to normal after the medication is withdrawn. Ten percent of the lupus population has this variation.
4. **Neonatal lupus** is a rare condition that arises at birth when the antibodies of a mother with lupus are passed to the newborn. (Don't be too alarmed, as the majority of women with lupus give birth to perfectly healthy babies.) For the majority of babies, these

symptoms resolve within six months without any permanent damage.

*As SLE accounts for the majority of lupus cases, this will be the focus of this book.

Lupus Doesn't Discriminate, Right?

There are significant differences in how lupus affects women of color compared to white women. Lack of equity in health care has made things worse for minority groups. Lupus is most common among individuals with African ancestry, less common among those with Hispanic or Asian ancestry, and least common among those with Caucasian ancestry.[4] Women of color often experience more severe symptoms, get diagnosed at a younger age, and face a higher risk of complications and death.[5]

Lupus is two to three times more common in Asian, African American, Hispanic/Latina, Native American, Alaska Native, and Pacific Islander women in the US.[6] Black women, in particular, have a death rate that is three times higher and are more likely to get a severe form of SLE at a young age.[7] It's important to note that lupus is the fifth leading cause of death for Black and Hispanic women aged 15 to 24.

Uniquely Lupus

Now we move on to the symptoms of lupus. How exactly does this disease show up?

Ah, ha. Gotcha. This is a trick question because there is no one way SLE (aka lupus) presents. It's rare to find another lupus patient who has the same symptoms as you. No two people are alike in their symptoms, like how people have unique fingerprints or their own sense of style. Some women have mild symptoms that are more annoying than anything, like a minor rash on their face. Others find themselves hospitalized regularly with multiple serious issues.

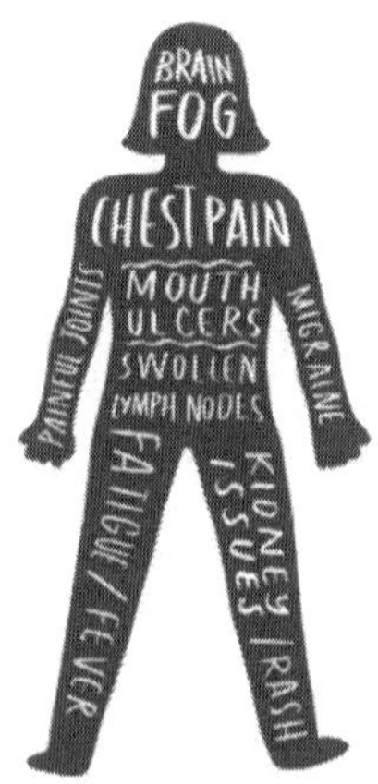

Symptoms on Full Display

One of the not-so-fun sides of lupus is that it can potentially affect every part of your body.

Yeah, you heard that right. This disease has the potential to ruin everything, including your lovely, shiny hair and cute piggy toes. Doesn't that suck? Here is a sampling of the ways lupus can impact your body:

- **Whole Body:** joint stiffness and/or swelling, arthritis,* fatigue, anemia (low iron), fever, nipple hair growth (just making sure you're paying attention, but this shouldn't happen), chest pain, weight gain/loss, blood clots, Raynaud's syndrome (fingers and toes in pain when cold), edema or swelling, sensitivity to light, digestive issues, kidney concerns, and cardiac issues.
- **Skin:** hair loss, patches of hair falling out, butter fly shaped rash on the face, sun sensitivity, red rash on the body, skin lesions, scaly rash, bruising, wounds healing slowly.
- **Mouth:** dryness, mouth ulcers, tongue cuts, dental issues, gingivitis, and a unique mix of oral bacteria that correlates with disease activity.
- **Mental:** anxiety, depression, brain fog, headaches, migraines, seizures, and even more.

Phew. That is a giant pile of symptoms, and, if you can believe it, there are still many others.

*Did you see that arthritis is listed as a symptom of SLE? Let's talk about this for a second. Arthritis is described as the pain, stiffness, swelling, and/or redness you feel in your joints. It can be felt in large joints, like the knees and shoulders, and also in the small joints of the fingers and toes. Lupus is not a form of arthritis. Rather, arthritis is a symptom of lupus, and unfortunately, 95 percent of lupus patients experience it.

Most Commonly Felt

When it comes to symptoms, the most common ones that show up in the body are:

- **Fatigue:** This extreme tiredness affects 80 to 90 percent of people living with lupus. Notice the emphasis used here—extreme. This doesn't mean you're just a wee bit tired, like, "I'll just pop by Starbucks for an iced Frappuccino to boost me up." It means you are bone tired—like tired even after the-best-nap-of-your life tired.
- **Pain:** The sucky reality is that 90 to 95 percent of people with lupus suffer from muscle and/or joint pain and stiffness. It can be felt at specific locations, like the knees, or as a full body ache similar to the flu. Stiff, tender, sore, swollen, and painful joints are the hallmarks of the disease.
- **Rash:** A butterfly-shaped red rash on the face wrapping around the cheeks and up to the nose is the hallmark rash of lupus. For others, like me, a variety of rashes can appear across the face and body. Sun exposure can worsen the rash and make lupus symptoms stronger.
- **Fever:** Women with lupus may run low grade fevers (100 or below) consistently. Other people have higher fevers that come and go when in a flare.
- **Hair loss:** Hair loss comes with SLE. Eek, not the hair too, you say. You may have extra hair loss in a flare—not like, "Oh, let me pull this random hair off my shirt," but more like a hundred or more strands each day.
- **Chest pain:** Inflammation in the heart and lungs causes chest pain. This pain, called pleuritis, feels sharp when you take a deep breath, cough, sneeze, or laugh. It may also make it harder to breathe.

- **Swelling:** When fluid builds up in the body, it usually causes swelling in the feet, ankles, legs, and eyelids. It can happen in other parts of the body too. This swelling can also be a sign of a kidney problem.
- **Anemia:** About half of the people who have lupus will have anemia. This is a condition in which inflammation keeps the body from using its stored iron.
- **Ulcers:** These painful ulcers are commonly found in the mouth or nose but can even show up in your vagina. It's like a little volcano that erupts, spewing hot lava of pain in the process.

Pay Attention

Don't ignore any symptoms, no matter how weird they feel or whether they were passed over by your doc. This means swollen lymph nodes, excessive fatigue, or many other things that just feel off. Trust your instincts. If something feels wrong, it may just be wrong. Keep digging until you get an answer to what's going on with you.

Your Future with Lupus

Now, let's address the question that's probably been weighing on your mind since receiving your diagnosis. It's a question that often prompts immediate googling, right after "What is lupus?" It's the burning question that many with lupus ask themselves: "Is this disease going to kill me?"

For the majority of people, lupus is not fatal. Phew! Take a breath. More people are living longer and healthier lives with lupus than ever before. In fact, 80 to 90 percent of people who have this autoimmune disease will likely live a normal life.

Not so fast, though. Chronic inflammation can lead to major problems that can change or shorten a person's life, such as kidney damage or failure, problems with blood clotting, strokes, or heart attacks. In fact, cardiovascular disease and heart attacks are the main causes of death in people with SLE.

What Factors Most Impact Lupus?

The most important things that affect health outcomes for many diseases, including lupus, are the social factors of health, such as financial stability, employment, access to and quality of education, neighborhood and living environment, social support, and access to health care.[8] Financial struggles increase the risk of death for people with lupus due to the disease and its complications. This is primarily due to the inability to get the medical care needed.

Individual factors that can make lupus symptoms worse are stress; not getting enough sleep; being alone; not being able to move around; PTSD, depression; anxiety; a history of sexual, physical, or emotional abuse; a person's coping method; a person's feelings about their disease (like anger, fear, or not being able to accept it); and beliefs about medications and vaccines. Also, not taking medicines and/or not following a doctor's orders can greatly impact one's lupus negatively.[9]

Reflections

- Lupus can affect any part of the body, is hard to diagnose, and remains incurable.
- There are four kinds of lupus, with SLE being the most widespread.
- When it comes to race, lupus certainly doesn't play fair.
- The most common signs are pain, tiredness, fever, rashes, and hair loss.

2

Lupus: Life's Unexpected Plot Twist

The body has great potential, but most people don't trust it.

—Andrew Weil, MD

For almost a decade, I questioned my first autoimmune diagnosis of Sjogren's. Sure, my mouth and eyes were a bit dry, but this didn't explain the constant mouth ulcers, the throbbing pain that began in my knees and moved its way up to my fingers and hands, or the low platelets and white blood cell count. Something was up. Deep down, I knew it was lupus, but it hadn't been confirmed.

During the COVID pandemic, I reached a new level of shittiness. My brain was foggy, and my mind was so forgetful. My throbbing knees kept me up at night, migraines kept me inside the house, and piles of hair were falling out. My rheumatologist referred me to a lupus specialist because I was now too sick for her to treat me, but I had to wait six months for an appointment. This wait was just like my attempts at Zumba: painful and scary.

Since help wasn't coming quickly enough for me, I took my health into my own hands and found a rheumatologist with only a two-month delay. I went to see her, and I was officially diagnosed with lupus. I started taking Plaquenil and thought that lupus would chill out and I'd start feeling like my old self again. I was so wrong about this!

These days, I straddle the line between "I'm okay" and "I'm totally not okay." Many days are good for me because I have a strong base of healthy habits that I can draw on, but that doesn't mean I'm immune to everything lupus throws at me. Quite the contrary. There are times that are downright shitty and scary, and I have to focus on just getting through the day.

This chapter plunges into the wacky world of lupus challenges. Get ready to uncover why lupus is a mischievous little troublemaker that loves to hide from diagnosis, leaving doctors scratching their heads. We'll spill the beans on lupus treatment strategies and what the research says about what causes lupus. (Brace yourself for the shocking revelation that, nope, you can't pin your lupus on eating gluten.)

Diagnosis

A lupus diagnosis is not as simple as you might imagine. One of the biggest challenges in diagnosing lupus is that there isn't a specific test that says, "Yep, you have lupus" or "Phew, you don't." To receive a diagnosis of lupus, a person must have at least four of the following eleven symptoms, according to the American College of Rheumatology:

- a butterfly rash on the cheeks
- rash on the face, arms, neck, or torso
- sensitivity to the sun
- recurring mouth or nose ulcers
- stiffness, swelling, and/or pain in the joints
- inflammation of the lungs or around the heart
- abnormalities in the urine, like protein
- nervous system problems, such as seizures
- problems with blood, such as anemia or reduced platelets
- lab tests that show increased autoimmune activity
- a positive result from an antinuclear antibodies (ANA) blood test

Lupus can show up in many different ways, so it may take a while for a doctor to figure out what's wrong. A physician may suspect lupus, but it might be the case where you don't have enough symptoms to make a diagnosis. In this case, the doctor will likely keep a close eye on you, checking in at regular intervals and ordering more tests as needed.

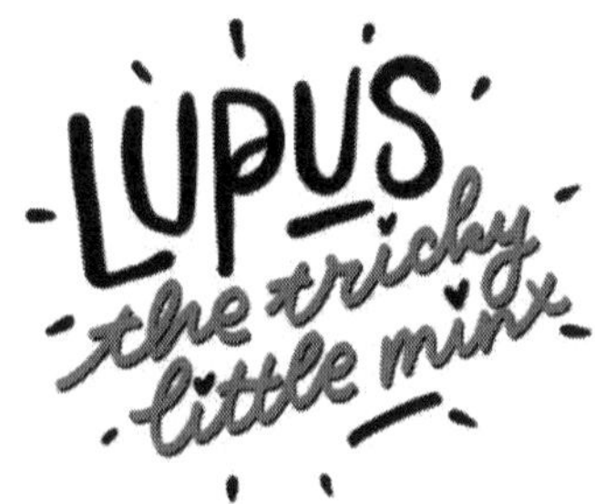

Lupus, the Tricky Little Minx

One out of every seven people who have lupus receives the wrong diagnosis, illustrating how difficult it can be to properly identify the condition. A few of the many reasons why this is true include:

- Lupus is difficult to diagnose because of the wide variety of symptoms, degrees of severity, and organ involvement.
- Lupus is called "the great imitator" because its symptoms can be like those of other conditions like fibromyalgia, hypothyroidism, and bacterial infections.
- For some people, symptoms come and go. Others might have a slow progression, where they first experience one symptom and others develop over time.
- Autoimmune diseases can progress in stages, and an early stage of one disease can resemble the advanced stage of another. This can lead to a diagnosis that keeps changing as the disease progresses.
- Having lupus and other diseases together can make it harder to figure out what's wrong.

Now you can begin to see why it can take up to six years to receive a correct lupus diagnosis. It also explains why your rheumatologist needs to be both a physician and Nancy Drew.

A delay in medical care during this time could permanently jeopardize your health. This creates a real internal shitstorm when combined with the general difficulty of diagnosing lupus, the prevalence of misdiagnoses, and the unknowns associated with this condition.

Invisible Side of Lupus

Lupus is called an "invisible" illness, which means that you cannot tell if someone has SLE just by looking at them. Because the symptoms cannot be seen, this can lead to misunderstandings, wrong ideas, and judgments from others. This is why you may hear "But you look so good" from a well-meaning friend.

And let me tell you, just because you don't have a cast or a bandage doesn't mean you're not hurting like a motherfucker. Unfortunately, people sometimes judge others solely by what they see. Have you ever known someone who seems confused when they see a person park in a handicapped spot who doesn't appear to be disabled? As you and I both know, when it comes to lupus, there's more than meets the eye.

Women Be Faking It

Because of the misunderstandings that come with this invisible illness, women with lupus often fake it, pretending that they feel better than they actually do. Acting like their bodies are doing fine, thank you very much. Concealing that lupus has maxed out their credit cards with co-pays, prescriptions, and a host of attempted remedies in an effort to heal. But in reality, they're suffering in silence.

Lupus Treatments

The ultimate goal of lupus treatments is to control symptoms, decrease organ damage, improve quality of life, and prevent, limit, and stop flares. **The best outcome for lupus is to have low disease activity or be in a state of remission.** It's the holy grail of lupus to be both pain free and symptom-free, and that's what everyone is searching for and praying for.

Would you believe me if I told you that the FDA has only approved three therapies to treat lupus in the last seventy years? The type of treatment your rheumatologist will offer depends on the symptoms you experience. This is because there's no cure for lupus, so the best they can do is manage what you are going through. Although there are only a few officially approved medications, rheumatologists use an arsenal of different treatments to manage lupus. Because symptoms can change frequently and treatments can have bad side effects, your rheumatologist may recommend a combination of ways to manage your SLE. Also, know that the treatments and medications you begin upon diagnosis will most likely not be the ones you continue with during your lifetime.

It took me a long time to find the mental strength to start taking the drugs my body desperately needed. When my rheumatologist first recommended medication, I stubbornly refused, afraid of admitting that my body had any weakness that I couldn't control. I pretended to be healthy and capable despite the pain I was experiencing. If you had offered up ashwagandha or some gnarly root from a bush in Ecuador, I would have been so game to give it a try. However, as the pain became unbearable, I finally understood the risks of my inaction and started taking the medications, knowing I had subjected my body to prolonged inflammation. The long-term damage remains uncertain, but it's a burden I must bear, even if it shortens my life. I made the best decisions I could with the knowledge I had, even though it wasn't enough.

I'm not here to tell you to take that medication your rheumatologist suggested—or not take it. I'm here to tell you that **you are in control of your health and need to be an active participant in your care** and have an open, honest discussion with your rheumatologist about what treatments are best for you.

Don't Stop

Do not stop taking your medication without talking to your doctor, even if you feel like it isn't working yet or if you don't like the side effects. And when you feel oh-so-fine, continue on your medications. Some drugs take months to make a positive impact. Other prescriptions work on a cellular level that you can't possibly see. Don't stop your medications simply to shove bee pollen up your nose after reading an article touting its benefits. Consult your doctor before making any prescription changes.

Sorry to get all yelly at ya, but this is serious stuff! People do not always take their meds, either because they forget or because they don't want to. This makes it hard for them to get the best care and affects how their bodies respond.

Keep in mind, too, that taking prescription medications does not mean you should abandon all other aspects of your health, like getting enough sleep and moving your body each day, as these are vital pieces of your overall health puzzle. There's room for a multipronged approach to managing your lupus. You can collaborate with your doctor, follow their recommendations, and find integrated ways to help maintain and grow your health.

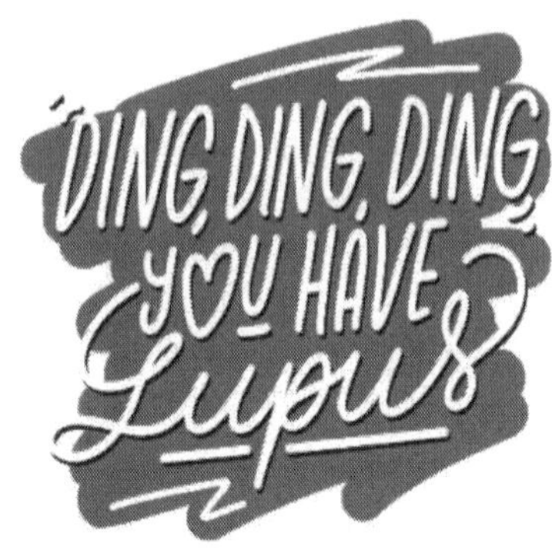

Who's to Blame for Lupus?

When you first receive a lupus diagnosis, you might wonder why and how you got it.

Can you blame it on your parents?

Can you blame it on a low-carb diet?

Can you blame it on all of those mean thoughts you had in high school?

Feel free to politely but firmly roll your eyes and extend your middle finger at anyone who tries to convince you that lupus is a result of sleeping with your socks on or forgetting to eat your vegetables. There is nothing you did to cause your lupus. You are not a bad person, and you are not at fault. Even though you may have angrily scrubbed the toilet with your brother's toothbrush at the age of thirteen (yes, I really did this), karma isn't getting back at you with lupus. **You are not being punished. You are not to blame for having lupus in your life. Lupus can happen to the best of human beings, including you. Lupus is not your fault!**

So, what actually causes lupus? Well, the truth is, the medical community doesn't know exactly what brings it on. It's like trying to figure out why some people are left-handed or why some people think pineapple belongs on pizza. There are definitely some genetic and environmental factors at play, but it's still a bit of a mystery.

Genetic predisposition

According to the Lupus Foundation of America, no single gene or group of genes has been proven to cause lupus, although there are some associated gene variations. Researchers have identified well over a hundred gene variations that are linked to lupus. A gene variation is a difference seen in our DNA sequence. It explains why one sibling has darker hair, why you have that cute dimple in your left cheek, and why B+ is your blood type. Genes influence who gets lupus and how severe it will be for that person. The more variations you inherit, the higher your chances of developing the disease. But there's more to it than your genes.

One theory is that certain viruses or infections can trigger lupus in people who are already genetically predisposed to it. It's like your immune system was just fine and dandy, minding its own business, and then one day it just snapped.

The point is, you can have gene variations for lupus, but these genes can remain turned off and dormant for all of your life if you are that fortunate. And most of the people born with these gene variations do not develop lupus. Lucky ducks! But when certain factors show up, they can flip the lupus switch to "on."

The worst kind of inheritance

The majority of people with lupus have no known relatives with this disease. Still, if you have an immediate family member with lupus, you are more likely to develop it when paired with a particular environmental trigger (more on this later). This is because environmental factors can damage cells, and then genetic inheritance comes into play.

About 5 percent of all kids whose parents have lupus will also get it.[10] Donald Thomas, Jr., MD, author and rheumatologist, stated that "if a mother has SLE, her daughters have as much as a 10 percent chance of developing SLE, while only 2 percent of her sons will develop lupus."[11] In twin studies, when one identical twin has lupus, there's a 24 to 66 percent chance the other twin will develop it as well. So science knows that genes are clearly involved, but there's more to this equation that hasn't been proven yet.[12] [13] Unfortunately, no genetic test can predict the risk of this disease.

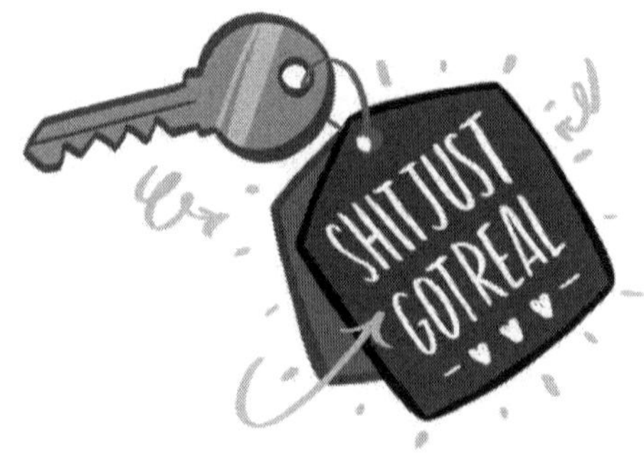

Female hormones

Hormones play a role in the development of lupus. Think of them as text messages your body receives that say, "Hey, send me more of that stress hormone because I'm about to go through a breakup." These hormones are quite powerful.

Sex hormones, in particular, are important with lupus. Estrogen is a hormone that helps keep your brain, bones, heart, and reproductive system healthy. While both genders have estrogen, females' levels are typically much higher. This is certainly true during menstruation and pregnancy. High estrogen levels may be the reason why women's immune systems are typically stronger, which is a good thing most of the time. But high estrogen can get a woman into trouble when her immune system goes into an overactive response and brings on lupus. This explains why SLE is typically diagnosed during women's childbearing years.

Lupus risk factors

Watch out for crafty lifestyle and environmental culprits that can pull a fast one and contribute to lupus, though they only account for a small part of the disease's overall risk. Researchers are actively trying to learn more about possible triggers for the onset or progression of the disease because lupus remains a mystery, but here's what's known so far.

1. Exposure to **silica dust** is a hazard in certain careers like construction, stone masonry, and ceramics. It increases the risk of SLE and other autoimmune diseases, but questions still exist about how exactly it causes these diseases.[14]
2. **Smoking**, including vaping, fills your body with harmful toxins. It's an addictive habit that is extremely unhealthy— please get

help with this right away. This also pertains to second hand smoke. Do everything possible to stay away from this.

3. **Infections**, like Epstein-Barr virus (EBV), have been linked to the development of SLE and other autoimmune diseases, but the exact mechanisms are not fully understood.[15] EBV is the virus that causes mononucleosis and lies dormant in the body for years. Cytomegalovirus (try saying that name out loud) is another common herpesvirus that is associated with autoimmunity, especially in people who are genetically predisposed.

There is a need for more research into the possible links between solvents, pesticides, heavy metals, air pollution, ultraviolet light, and SLE. Many studies have also shown that the toxic chemicals we are exposed to every day can affect our immune system at the cellular level.[16] Just because mold, toxic gas, pesticides, and too much sun haven't been proven with 100 percent certainty to trigger lupus, use some common sense here. They aren't good for anyone, especially not people with chronic inflammatory diseases. Do what you can to limit your exposure to these factors.

Reflections

- Lupus can be quite challenging to diagnose for a variety of reasons and can take up to six years to be confirmed.
- The invisibility of some aspects of lupus makes it harder for others to understand what you're going through.
- Rheumatologists treat lupus based on the symptoms that show up.
- Lupus is not your fault, but science still does not know exactly what causes it.

3

Flare and Flare Care (Say That Three Times Quickly)

Always remember that prevention is the most important form of medicine.

—Lisa See, *Lady Tan's Circle of Women*

My worst flare to date occurred while writing this book. It started with growing exhaustion, and then my most hated, much dreaded leg pain returned. It feels like I've run a full marathon (although I never have) and I get shooting pain and tingling sensations up and down my legs. These symptoms hung around for a few weeks as I tried to rest more and control my stress, but I only became more withdrawn and irritable. When a new symptom showed up, I was officially scared because I knew inflammation had reached my brain. I woke up one day so dizzy that I could only look straight ahead. It felt like my brain was continuously being shocked, and I seriously thought I was having a stroke. I was terrified. I canceled all meetings and events and refused to see anyone or take phone calls from friends. I stopped writing because the words wouldn't come out of my brain. I thought life wasn't worth it if I had to live like this. I was completely disconnected from reality, lost in a deep, black void.

To top it all off, a month into my worst flare, I got bangs. Who the hell gets bangs at a time like this? I should have anticipated the extra energy required by a complex hairstyle. If I didn't have enough energy to pick myself up off the bed, there was no way I would wrangle those wiry hairs sticking out of my head into something that looked somewhat decent. Not only was I in terrible pain, but I had added more stress to my routine than I needed.

After six weeks, I finally went to my rheumatologist for steroids and had an MRI because my brain was so badly screwed up. What took me so long, you ask? You'd think I knew better; after all, I was writing a freaking book on this. Clearly, I didn't. I was in denial for a while, hoping the flare would resolve. Then, I convinced myself that taking a steroid would be worse than the flare (it actually wasn't), and I didn't want to bother my doctor. With all of this, I was so wrong, and I hurt myself by allowing the inflammation to get to my vital brain.

So, the moral of my story is this: If you're going through a tough SLE phase, maybe hold off on the complicated haircuts (or other big decisions) for a while. And don't be afraid to get a hold of your rheumatologist early on when they're truly needed.

It's also possible to prepare yourself for the ups and downs of lupus flares, where your body may decide at any moment to host a party of strange symptoms. Understanding yourself and your triggers is crucial for reducing their impact on your life. When you develop deeper flare self-awareness, you can work on ways to lessen your symptoms and short circuit the flares early on. And when flares do show up, you don't have to be totally miserable. There are steps you can take to feel better quicker. Grab your notepad, put on your detective hat, and let's crack the code of a flare management strategy.

Understanding a Flare

An extra sucky part of having lupus is when your pain and symptoms worsen and a flare comes on. A flare amplifies your normal level of pain exponentially. For example, if your normal pain level is 5 out of 10, it could reach 9 during a flare-up. The intense symptoms can make you feel like you have the flu, COVID, or both. A flare can range in intensity from unpleasant to potentially fatal, as in the case of severe organ damage.

Flares are hard to predict (but not impossible) and can have a big impact on all parts of your life. The good news is that flares only last a few days to a few weeks—occasionally a few months. It won't go on forever, even though it feels otherwise.

Your goal is to have as few flares as possible because less SLE activity means less lupus damage and a healthier you.

While each person has their own unique flare characteristics, the most common symptoms are:

- painful joints (that may or may not be swollen)
- fatigue that transforms into extreme exhaustion
- brain fog
- mouth or nose sores
- fever (not due to an infection)
- hair loss
- new or worsening rash

If you do all that you can to reduce the flare symptoms on your own and still cannot find relief after several days, contact your rheumatologist. If your case is not urgent, they will let you know and prioritize it accordingly.

Another, often quicker, option is to utilize your primary care provider (PCP). My PCP likes to remind me that they serve on the care team for patients with autoimmune diseases.

Warning: Get Help

There are certain new flare symptoms that should not be ignored. They can be very serious and warrant an immediate trip to the ER and include:

1. Numbness on one side of the body or face. Fatigue, confusion, motor dysfunction, or speech impairment may accompany this.
2. Sudden chest pain or shortness of breath
3. Pain, swelling, and possibly redness of the calf area
4. Weakness of an arm, leg, or side of the face
5. A severe headache, like the worst headache ever, especially if coupled with nausea, fever, weakness, or numbness in the arm, leg, or face
6. Severe stomach pain combined with other symptoms such as fever, nausea, vomiting, or blood in the stool
7. Blurred vision, with or without fever, headache, or blindness in one eye
8. Swelling of the ankles/feet, foamy urine, change in color of urine. These are all signs of a lupus nephritis attack, and you don't get back kidney function once damaged.

IF TACOS CAN FALL APART
AND STILL BE
AMAZING,
SO CAN YOU

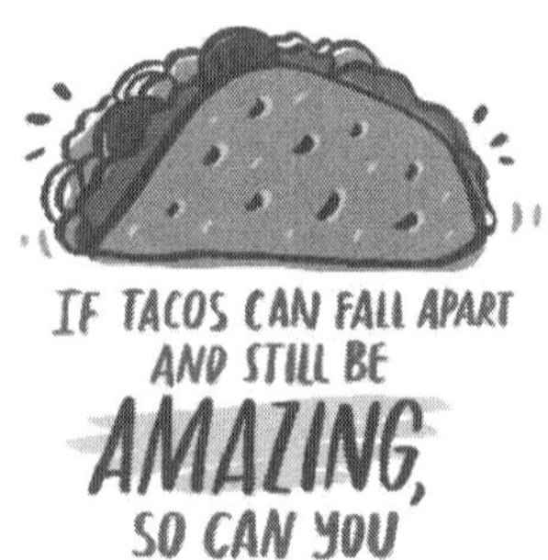

Plan for Flare Relief

There are ways you can stay in control of your symptoms and pain, even during the hardest times, by developing strategies for coping. A flare management plan helps you reduce the frequency, severity, and length of your flare-ups. It also gives you tools get yourself through these tough times, which will give you more confidence in your ability to deal with flare-ups in the future.

It's important to note that while these strategies may gradually reduce the intensity of pain, they won't give you instant relief. But over time, they will help you manage your pain, stay active, and feel better.

What's on This Plan?

Your flare management plan is based on what works for you, and your SLE and has two parts:

1. A plan to avoid a flare
2. A plan for what to do when a flare happens.

Step 1: Identify Triggers

The first step is to think about what can cause a flare-up for you. Rheumatologist Alexa Meara, MD, says, "Any changes in your environment can cause an inflammatory reaction." This means that any time you adjust your normal routine, you bump up your risk of inflammation and the chance of a flare. This helps to explain why working on a mentally taxing project or moving to a new home could be triggering.

Maybe you've noticed a connection between flares and something you did or ate, how you moved, how much sleep you got, or a host of other factors. A flare-up might also happen after a big life change or stressful event. Or maybe you've experienced a flare-up for seemingly no reason, but it just popped up on its own like a big zit on your chin.

Most flares-up don't just randomly appear. Your body has certain sensitivities or triggers. The most common include:

- increasing stress
- exhaustion
- sun exposure
- infection and/or illness
- stopping medicine or making changes to it

Really get to know your body. Pay careful attention to how you feel in the AM and PM, mentally, spiritually, physically, and emotionally. Be so in tune with your body that you're able to connect the dots when that lack of water yesterday made you slightly constipated today or when arguing with your friend caused you to miss out on quality sleep. Keep a journal of how you feel, or make notes on your phone. **A flare can sneak up on you if you're not in tune with your habits and routines**. This is exactly what you want to avoid.

The things that cause your flare-ups are your red flags. They stop you from feeling good. Now think about what you can do to avoid triggers and head off the flare. These are your green flags, and most likely, they are enjoyable for you too. Here are a few examples for you:

Red Flag

Going out late to drink with girlfriends leaves you extra tired, dehydrated, and cranky the next day.

Green Flag

You choose to drink two cups of water before going out, limit yourself to one drink, and come home by 10 p.m.

Red Flag

When a big deadline is looming, you prioritize it over everything else, forgoing nutritious meals and your fave cycling class. You're wiped out after work and spend all evening vegging out on the couch.

Green Flag

At the start of the day, you set your work priorities. You will eat lunch away from your computer, get up from your desk every 1.5 hours for a bit, and stop working at 6 p.m.

Now it's your turn. Think through the things that wear you out, bring on stress, or cause you pain. Write down your red flags below. Then decide how you can counter a red flag with an action that lowers or removes the pain.

Your Red Flag

____

____

____

____

Your Green Flag

____

____

____

____

Your Red Flag

____

____

____

____

Your Green Flag

____

____

____

____

Step 2: Create a Plan

Now that you've got a plan in place to keep those pesky flare-ups at bay, it's important to be ready for those times when they still sneak up on you. Take a moment to think about the things that really help you manage your pain and bring you some much needed comfort. Keep in mind, too, the things that don't really help when you're in the midst of a flare-up.

What helps in a flare? (Taking rest breaks. Calling Tina, my SLE friend. Using a heat pad.)

____

____

____

____

What's something you love to do that loves you right back? (Walking my dog. Reading a juicy romance. Iced coffee.)

____

____

____

____

What doesn't help? (Too much sugar, bingeing on Instagram, or lying on the couch.)

____

____

____

____

Once you've had a good think, grab a pen and jot down ten practical steps you can take whenever a flare-up strikes. These steps should be your go to moves. So, take your time and create your very own flare-up management plan.

My Flare-Up Management Plan

1.____
2.____
3.____
4.____
5.____
6.____
7.____
8.____
9.____
10.____

When your body is in a flare, preparing a healthy, nutritious meal just isn't happening. Like, I don't have energy to take a shower, yet I'm supposed to make a large salad with ten chopped ingredients? No way!

It's normal to crave high-fat and high-sugar foods under pressure or in a flare. As hard as it is, don't give in to temptation and eat like shit. You will only feel worse and be more likely to react badly.

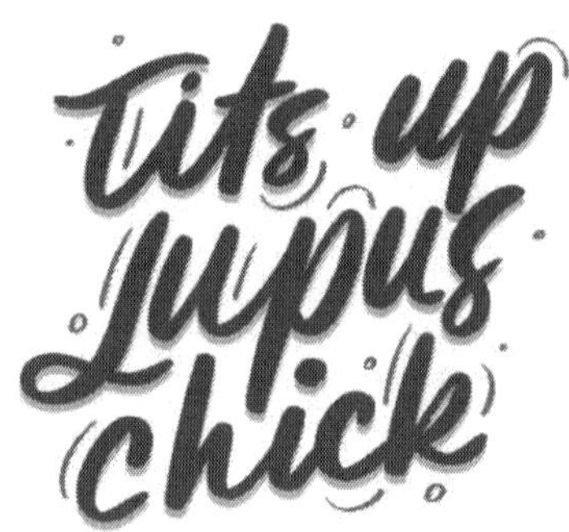

When under stress, your body uses up nutritional resources that have been saved, resulting in the need for even more vitamins and nutrients. To counter this, eat fruits like kiwis, lemons, oranges, and grapefruits; almonds; and legumes that fill the body back up with essential nutrients.

Additional ways to use food to help with a flare include:

- Cut down on the time you spend making meals so you have more time to take care of yourself.
- Make meals ahead of time and place them in the freezer. When a flare happens, simply defrost the food and eat it. Most foods can last up to a year in the freezer. Soups like minestrone and lasagna freeze really well, as do avocados. (Surprising, huh?)

- Create a list of foods and restaurants that you enjoy. When your family or friends want to help, they can buy food from this list.
- Be careful not to eat too much sodium, potassium, and fat when you're flaring. This just means extra work for your hard-pressed kidneys.
- Keeping crappy food around when you're already feeling crappy is a bad idea. Throw it away.

More Tips to Get You through a Flare

Prioritize what's important: When you are starting to feel run down, it's time to put your energy toward what's truly important. Think through your day and choose to focus on the most vital things and let other people or tasks wait. Avoid anything that is draining, stressful, or that you just don't want to do (unless it's work, because that money is needed).

Lean on others: Call a girlfriend or loved one who is (1) compassionate and (2) willing to truly listen to you. If you don't have any friends like this, find an online lupus community where you feel heard and supported.

Change up your environment: It's hard to get dressed and function in a flare. That's why staying at home and hanging out in your sweats feels good. But changing up what's around you can actually help ease the pain. When you're in a new space (whether that's a coffee shop or walking in a different area), your brain has to put energy into processing all of this new stuff, and this means there's less energy available to make you feel like shit.

Mantra: A mantra is a powerful way to get through difficult times. Mine is *"This too shall pass,"* and it reminds me that everything is temporary—even when it feels otherwise. Want some examples? Try out one of these babies:

- I'm dope AF!
- No matter what comes up, I love and trust my body!
- I love myself!
- It's all going to work out!
- I am doing a fucking amazing job!

Reflections

- Understanding why you flare is essential for managing SLE and living a good life.
- You can reduce the number and severity of flare-ups by figuring out your triggers and staying away from them.
- Eat extra healthy when in a flare because it will help the body recover quicker.
- With patience, persistence, and a plan of attack, you may even be able to feel decent on a daily basis. Shocker, but totally doable.

4

Finding a Kick-Ass Rheumatologist

I refuse to settle for something less than great. And if it takes a lifetime, then that's how long I'll wait.

—Dolly Parton

My quest for a decent rheumatologist has been a wild ride. More practices have turned me down than I can count, and two of the last three rheumatology clinics I visited closed. Can I catch a break, please?

But hope arose when I finally got referred to Dr. Saira Sheikh at the University of North Carolina. The only catch? I'd have to wait six months. But hey, good things come to those who wait, and I was willing to do so for the amazing SLE care that I deserve and ended up receiving.

Let me tell you, finding the right rheumatologist is crucial! It's like finding the perfect pair of shoes—you need someone who's going to support you, keep you comfortable, and help you strut your stuff. When you're dealing with SLE issues, having the right doctor on your side can make all the difference. And let's be real, we all know how important it is to have a trusted rheumatologist. Someone who truly listens to your concerns, understands the impact lupus has, and doesn't make you feel like you're crazy—I mean, is that too much to ask for?

In this chapter, you will learn how to get the care you need and deserve, because why wouldn't you want the best, most amazing rheumatologist in your corner? You'll learn how to locate a good rheumatologist and what to consider as you welcome this doctor into your lupus world. If you've ever considered participating in a lupus trial, we'll talk about that too.

Say It Ain't So: Lack of Rheumatologists

My hunt for a good rheumatologist is not a unique one. You've probably had a similar experience, as the entire rheumatology medical workforce in the United States is in jeopardy.

The Centers for Disease Control (CDC) estimates that at least 24 million people have an autoimmune disease, and an estimated 91 million people live with joint pain yet are not formally diagnosed. And there are only 5,595 rheumatologists available to care for these millions of people who need help.[17] In ten years, roughly half of all rheumatologists in the United States will be retired, and there won't be enough new doctors to fill this void. And those with autoimmune issues will feel this pain on many levels.

The long wait to see a rheumatologist makes things even more difficult.[18] The national average wait time is four weeks. From my research, the wait time ranges from two to eight months. Also, you can't just self-refer to a rheumatologist; a PCP or other qualified expert must do so.

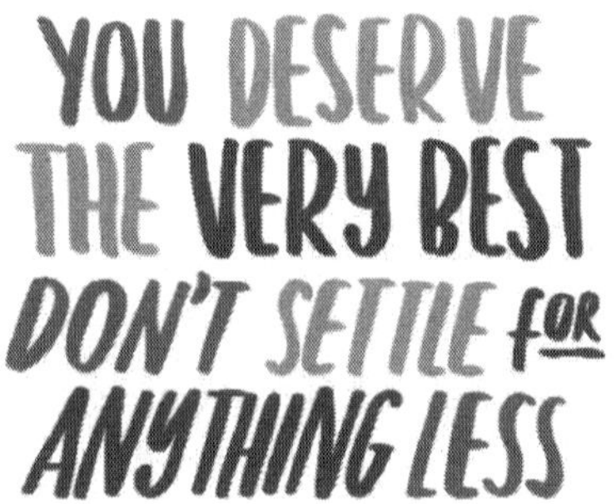

How to Score an Awesome Rheumatologist

First things first, do your research. Pester your PCP about their favorite rheumatologist and why they're so great, then crosscheck your insurance for coverage. If you've got a friend who's going through a similar autoimmune struggle, hit them up for some tips on local sources.

Hey, if you happen to have a doctor or pharmacist in the family, milk that connection for all it's worth.

Having a hard time finding someone? Try expanding your search to the next largest city to see if any new results emerge. If you have a local university or college with a medical program, look at their rheumatology program. Also, consider contacting a national lupus organization for help locating a rheumatologist.

If you can afford it and your insurance coverage makes this possible, you may even look for a provider out of state. This option could be appealing if there is a highly regarded rheumatologist you want to see or if cutting-edge care is available. For example, if you need help with the neuropsychiatry of lupus, you might look to a well-known rheumatology practice like the Johns Hopkins Lupus Center.

Dig Deeper

Once you've found a rheumatology practice, it's time to dig deeper. Read all of the Google and Yelp reviews with some skepticism. After all, you know people are more likely to write a review when they are angry and feel slighted.

Beyond reviews, some key things to look for include a rheumatologist's experience with lupus, board certification in rheumatology and internal medicine, hospital affiliations, and any past medical claims or malpractice lawsuits. You'll also want to consider any recent publications or research they've done in the field.

Skipping the Line

If you've called a practice and the wait time is super long for new patients, don't give up hope. There are still things you can do to be seen sooner. The first tip is to ask if they have a cancellation list you can be placed on. Would seeing an extender (a nurse practitioner or physician's assistant) get you an appointment faster? Try calling in each week (or every day if you're feeling feisty) to see if there are new patient openings in their schedule. Finally, plead with the person on the phone, asking, "What would you do if you were me?" and "What tips could you give me to be seen quicker?"

If your PCP feels your case is more urgent, they will alert the rheumatology practice about this. What typically happens is that the rheumatology practice will review your chart once it is received and determine the severity of your case. Try not to be offended if they say, "Nah, you don't seem that bad," and then tell you to wait five months for the first appointment.

First Visit

Before your first visit, write down all the questions you want to ask. It's easy to forget this in the moment, plus there's that brain fog thing making matters worse. During the appointment, think of it as an interview you're conducting. Does the rheumatologist look you in the eyes when speaking? Are your questions given the time and importance they deserve? Does the appointment feel rushed? Are your opinions and thoughts considered in the overall SLE care plan?

By the end of your appointment, ask these questions:

- Who's involved in your care team? (RN, nurse practitioner, etc.)
- What should you do in a flare?
- How are refills handled?
- How long does it take for messages and calls to be answered?

In the end, decide if you feel supported and comfortable with this doctor's care. If yes, awesome sauce. Continue on. If not, move on. You deserve the very best rheumatologist, and it may take some time to find this person.

Develop Your Doc Patient Relationship

Think of your relationship with your rheumatologist as a collaboration where there's equal give and take in order to find answers and create solutions. This empowers you to advocate for yourself and encourages your doctor to do their very best. To have this, trust and clear communication are essential. You'll need to be open and honest at each and every appointment. Don't just say what you think you should say. If you're scared about your chest pain, tell them and admit the fact that you're vaping. Be as descriptive as possible. Your rheumatologist cannot help you if they don't understand the full scope of what's going on. Their job is to listen to your pain and symptoms and figure out what is wrong in order to give you solutions that fit your needs.

If your doctor's explanations and responses are unclear or unhelpful, let them know. This feedback will encourage your doctor to listen and continue to offer help. If you need more information or didn't understand something, share that too. Give your doctor the chance to clarify, to make sure you're both on the same page.

Your Doc Is Human Too. Promise.

Remember that your rheumatologist is an imperfect human being, just like you. You can assume that your doctor tries their best to keep you healthy. If you don't feel like this, it sounds like it's time to get a new rheumatologist. Too often, we forget this and expect our doctor to know exactly what to do and remember everything about us. During a visit with my rheumatologist, I was reminded of this when she came in upset after losing a young SLE patient. The phone call informing her of the woman's death had just come in, and she had to immediately make her way across the hospital to see me. She needed time alone to deal with the pain, but I was there.

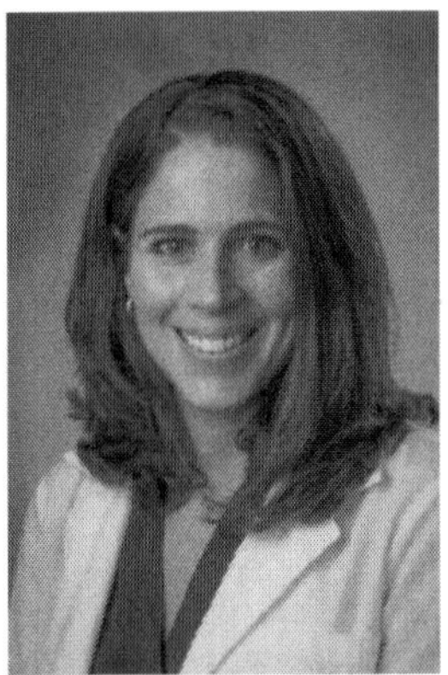

Interview with a Rheumatologist

Dr. Jennifer Rogers is an assistant professor of medicine, director of the Duke Lupus Clinic, director of the IJ Rheumatology Clinic, and co-director of the Duke Lupus Registry and Biorepository. Along with her colleagues at Duke, she developed the type 1 and type 2 SLE symptom models in order to capture the full spectrum of lupus symptoms, integrate the patient's perspective with science, and improve the delivery of lupus care. Here, Dr. Rogers shares helpful advice for women newly diagnosed with lupus:

1. **Build a Trustworthy Care Team**: Find a rheumatologist, primary care physician, and other care team members whom you genuinely trust, like an ophthalmologist if you take Plaquenil because of the potential side effects, or a nephrologist if you have kidney nephritis. Cultivating relationships based on open communication, mutual understanding, and respect is so important. It takes commitment and openness from both sides to create a strong and supportive partnership.
2. **Share Your Experience:** Openly discuss your lupus journey with the important people in your life. By sharing your experiences, you allow them to learn from you, understand your challenges, and grow alongside you. Their support and empathy can make a significant difference in your overall well-being. At the same time, remember that hearing other people's lupus stories can help you learn more about your disease and how to deal with it.
3. **Give Yourself Grace:** It's important to give yourself permission to prioritize self-care. It's okay to cut back on activities, rest when needed, and ask for help when necessary. Be kind to yourself and recognize that self-care is a vital part of managing lupus.
4. **Pace Yourself:** Lupus can be unpredictable, so it's crucial to pace yourself and listen to your body. Set your own limits and boundaries while striving for personal goals to improve your well-being. This may include focusing on techniques such as deep breathing, gentle movement, and acceptance of your condition.

Advance Yourself in a Lupus Trial

Have you ever thought about participating in a lupus clinical trial? By taking part in a trial, you will get fast access to the latest treatments and technologies for lupus while improving the lives of people with SLE and advancing our understanding of lupus—all worthwhile goals. To this day, I have participated in four different clinical trials, two of which were specifically for lupus. Even though I was uncertain at first, it made me feel good to be able to give something back to the lupus community, but I've also made steps toward improving my SLE.

There's a significant gender disparity in clinical trials that's worth mentioning here. Women only make up 41 percent of participants, even though we make up 51 percent of the population and 90 percent of the

SLE cases.[19] Simply put, we need more women and women from underrepresented groups to participate in order to ensure that clinical care and guidelines are truly representative of the SLE patient population as a whole. This shows that your involvement is crucial, regardless of your age, race, or background.

The benefits of being a participant are pretty cool. You have access to treatments before they are available to the general public. Plus, you'll have a more active role in your healthcare journey and contribute to the development of better SLE treatments in the future. Many participants are also paid for their time during the trial. Sure, there are risks involved, like potential side effects or the treatment not being more effective than what you're already receiving. And at times, trials can be a bit inconvenient and time consuming.

Consider observational/retrospective trials too. Many places have registry trials where they enroll patients, collect their data (questionnaires, lab work, DNA samples, biopsy samples, etc.), and then dig deep to analyze the data obtained. There is no risk to the participant, and it helps researchers learn more about lupus.

Now let's talk about the trial process. It's all about following protocols and staying informed. Before you sign up, they'll give you all the details about the study's purpose, your role, and any potential risks or side effects. It's like going on a date with no obligations, and you can back out at any time. During the trial, a team of experts will be closely monitoring you, just like your mom did during your rebellious teenage years. If anything goes wrong, they can shut it down in a flash. And don't worry: clinical trials aren't meant to replace your primary healthcare. They're more like a short-term fling, offering specific treatments for certain conditions. So, you'll keep seeing your doctor and taking your medications, and the research team will work alongside them to ensure your safety.

But here's an important challenge we need to tackle: a lack of racial diversity in clinical trials. It's crucial for better accuracy. Unfortunately, mistrust within the Black community prevents some individuals from participating due to historical mistreatment and ongoing healthcare disparities. We need to increase awareness, build trust, and promote inclusivity to overcome this hurdle.

Reflections

- Dig deep and don't stop until you uncover the best rheumatologist for you.
- The dwindling number of rheumatologists is concerning but still manageable.
- Developing a strong relationship with your doctor requires clear and honest communication.
- Clinical lupus trials need your contribution to make treatments more impactful.

5

Beyond the Finances, Drugs, and Gaslighting

Everything can be taken from a man but one thing: the last of the human freedoms—to choose one's attitude in any given set of circumstances, to choose one's own way.

—Viktor Frankl

When the pain became unbearable for me, I finally sought help. But instead of giving me the guidance I desperately needed, the doctor's dismissive words hit me hard. "You are not young anymore," he casually remarked, attributing my suffering to nothing more than age. Shit, I wasn't even forty yet. It was a crushing moment, feeling ignored and humiliated for daring to get the help I clearly needed. As he looked at me, I could tell he did not want to be there and that my problems did not matter. I mumbled thanks and got the hell out of there, carrying the weight of his ignorance and my own invisibility with me.

Here's the thing: he was completely wrong. I didn't just have one autoimmune disease; I had two. Thank you very much. To this day, I doubt that physician ever realized the impact of his actions or how invisible I felt under his care.

Upon reflection, I recognize that I was experiencing medical gaslighting. Maybe it was because I'm a woman, or perhaps he was just an insensitive jerk. Either way, I refuse to let my pain be invalidated. I stand here today as a wiser person, determined to shed light on the darkness of such experiences.

In this chapter, you'll delve into the issue of medical gaslighting and discover how to stand up for yourself when facing it. You'll learn when and how to seek a second opinion to ensure you receive the care you deserve. We'll also explore the financial impact of living with lupus, along with practical tips for managing your SLE money. Lastly, we'll review the spoon theory, a powerful metaphor that will underscore the importance of preserving your energy and resources. So, let's dive in.

Medical Gaslighting

Medical gaslighting occurs when a medical provider downplays a patient's concerns. It's when someone in power uses manipulation to make another person doubt their own judgment/sanity. This is like when a doctor tells you, "It's all in your head," and you're like, "Uh, no, it's not. It's in my body, which is attached to my head."

Medical gaslighting is a very real condition that has been happening for far too long. If you are a woman, a young woman, a woman of color, and/or part of the LGBTQA community, there's a high probability that you've experienced this once or twice. Hell, maybe many times.

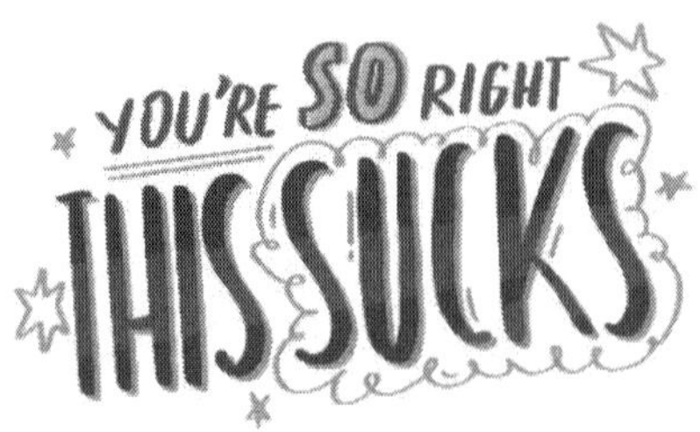

When a patient comes in, the provider looks at their race, sexual orientation, weight, socioeconomic status, and/or gender and forms an instant opinion, often without paying attention to the patient's problems and concerns. Plus, let's be real, sometimes doctors can be clueless when it comes to women's bodies and symptoms. Instead of admitting they don't know what's going on, they'll just brush it off and act like nothing's wrong.

How medical gaslighting may show up:

- You are interrupted, ignored, or not allowed to have a voice in the conversation.
- Your symptoms are minimized, downplayed, or blamed on something else.
- Your provider refuses to order labs or imaging to help with the diagnosis.
- You don't feel included in the decision-making process.
- You believe that your provider is manipulating, shaming, or belittling you.

Being overlooked, disregarded, or given the wrong diagnosis delays treatment, can permanently damage your health, and leads to unnecessary suffering. All in all, it's terribly wrong and hurtful.

What's a Girl to Do?

If you feel that you aren't being treated in the manner that you deserve, trust your gut. **You have every right to be heard and respected as a patient.** You also have the right to have your conditions, test results, medications, and treatments explained in a manner that makes sense to you. If this isn't happening, you can fire your rheumatologist, switch to a different doctor in that practice, or find a new one. Knowing that there is often a wait to see a new rheumatologist, be aware that you'll need to keep your current doctor in the meantime.

It's up to you to hold your doctor accountable. If you notice a disconnect in the conversation or feel unheard, take a pause and explain what you've noticed. As calmly as you can, state your concern, like, "I'm worried that my memory problems aren't being taken seriously. I want to talk more about this." If you didn't feel like your question was answered the first time, try asking it in a different way. For example, you might say, "When I walk, I now have a sharp pain in my right hip. Will you take a look at this? How can we deal with this?"

If your concern is still not addressed, you can file a complaint with the medical director at the medical practice. Most of the time, this will solve the problem to the point where you're satisfied. But if not, you can make a formal report against the physician with your local state medical board and also write a review online.

Getting a Second or Third Opinion

If you aren't getting what you need from your current physician, it's time to check out another option. It's common in the medical field to ask for this when it comes to big healthcare decisions.The majority of the time, your physician won't be offended that you've asked. If you do meet resistance, stand firm and know it's your right to get the very best care.

How would you know if and when to look for a second opinion? Look over the reasons below to see if any resonate with you:

- You don't trust your rheumatologist, or something feels off.
- You disagree with the diagnosis, or it's unclear.
- You can't decide between two treatment options.
- Other medical conditions complicate your care.
- A treatment or clinical trial is offered elsewhere.

The temporary guilt you may feel from pursuing another doc will go away once you feel confident with the new rheumatologist. Think of it this way: if this second opinion gives you peace of mind, then it's totally worth it. In the end, you have to live every day in that body of yours, so you need to make the best decision for yourself and fight for the best possible results.

How do you ask for a referral? Try this: "I'd like a referral to see Dr. X. Can your team process this for me?" It's simple and to the point. There is no need to explain more.

Financial Burden of Lupus

Let's be real, having lupus can be a real pain in the wallet. Did you know the average healthcare cost for someone with lupus is over $33,000 a year?[20] Even those with the mildest symptoms can have crazy-high medical bills, co-pays, and insurance fees. And don't even get me started on the indirect costs, like losing out on productivity and work. With 64 percent of Americans living paycheck to paycheck, a single flare-up or a new medical condition can really make a dent in your hard-earned savings.

Even though lupus can put a lot of stress on your finances, you can be proactive and find ways to lower medical expenses.

1. Get to know your insurance plan inside and out. Learn about your co-pays, co-insurance, and deductible limits. Call your insurance company for help if you're totally confused.
2. Whenever possible, stay in-network to save the most money. When you go out of network, your costs will be higher, sometimes astronomically higher.
3. Call your insurance plan to confirm estimated costs before scans, procedures, new medications, or surgeries.
4. If you are denied pharmacy coverage, don't just accept it. Fight it with an appeal. I was initially denied coverage for Benlysta. After speaking to my rheumatologist, she wrote a letter on my behalf, and the medication was approved.

Big Hospital Bills

After a hospitalization, request an itemized bill statement and check it line by line for charges. You won't want a hospital summary statement; the charges are not broken down here. According to Medical Billing Advocates of America, seven out of ten medical bills have some type of mistake. If there's a charge on the bill that looks unfamiliar, call the hospital to ask about it.

When facing a large hospital bill, a financial care counselor can help you arrange a payment plan with manageable monthly payments. As long as the hospital billing department sees that you are working to pay off your debt, they are more willing to make accommodations for you.

Consider asking for a bill discount. Do not feel bad about asking for this. Price adjustments are very common in our extremely overpriced medical system, and you may be able to score yourself some savings simply by asking.

There are hospital advocates and financial assistance programs out there to help you deal with the costs that come along with these large bills. Our health insurance plan had a great perk that helped with a costly emergency department bill. They provided us with an advocate who spoke on our behalf and lowered the bill by $4,000. If your plan doesn't offer this, you can pay an outside medical billing company to analyze your bills to find errors, overcharges, duplicate charges, and unreasonable charges.

Prescriptions

Let's talk about prescriptions, as they make up the majority of monthly healthcare expenses. Here are some ways to decrease your drug costs:

- Choose generic versions of your drugs. Ask your rheumatologist for their opinion before switching over if you've started on the brand name version.
- Price shop at local and online pharmacies because there can be big variations in pricing. For a 90-day supply of Plaquenil in the Raleigh area, the price ranged from $33 to $166 at our local pharmacies.
- Get a 90-day supply of your medication for bigger savings.
- Use a pharmacy savings card, like Good Rx or Well Rx, for deeper discounts. Sometimes these are better than your copays.
- Consider a patient assistance program (PAP) that can help lower or cover the drug costs for you. I use a PAP for Benlysta, a biologic, and my copays went from $200 a month to $0.

New Drugs

One of the main reasons why people struggle to take their medicines as prescribed is a lack of knowledge about the drugs and how to properly use them. It's time to take charge of your health by actively working with your doctor to understand why this new prescription is being suggested. Make sure to ask plenty of questions to learn more about the drug, what it is meant to treat, and exactly how it works.

Having answers to the following questions will help you feel more at ease with the suggested medication:

- What are the typical side effects, and which are concerning?
- How and when should you take the medication?
- When can you expect results?
- What should you avoid while taking this drug?
- Why is this drug being recommended?

Balancing Work and Lupus

Working with lupus can be tricky, especially when you can't predict when your symptoms will worsen or how bad you'll feel over time.

Whether or not to disclose your lupus diagnosis to your employer is a personal decision (and not a mandatory one) that depends on factors like your symptoms and job requirements. But telling your boss and coworkers about your condition can keep them informed and ready to help you, both now and in the future.

While many individuals with lupus can continue working with adjustments like flexible hours or telecommuting, it's important to communicate your needs to your employer and explore possible modifications to your work environment. Employers with fifteen or more workers are required by the Americans with Disabilities Act (ADA) to make reasonable accommodations for people with disabilities or chronic illnesses like lupus. These changes should not be hard to make or cost a lot of money. They can be things like a desk that is not near the window, a closer parking spot, or working in the afternoon instead of the morning, when the pain is the worst. A face-to-face meeting is a great way to begin this discussion on your accommodation needs and follow up on your request in writing for tracking purposes.

If there are work changes that could help you, you can ask your rheumatologist to write you a note about medically necessary alterations. Seeing an occupational therapist can also help because they can look at your job and figure out what changes or adjustments could be made.

If your lupus makes it too difficult for you to work, you may be eligible for Social Security Disability Insurance (SSDI) benefits. However, it's important to know that the application process for SSDI can be lengthy and often has a low success rate—a bummer indeed.

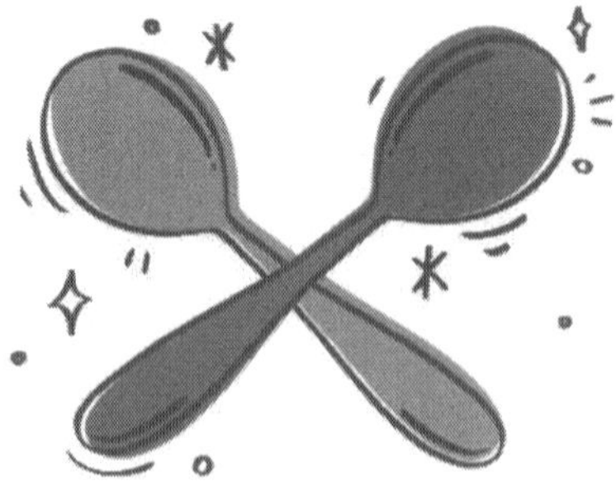

Enter the Spoons

Most healthy people can start their day with an unlimited amount of energy to do whatever the hell they desire without worrying about the effects of their actions. If they wear themselves out, they can rest up and feel fine and dandy the next day. But having lupus makes it harder to do this, especially when you have to carefully manage your daily activities to anticipate and accommodate your pain levels. That pain—and the logistics of managing it—can have an impact on your mental and physical bandwidth.

How does the Spoon Theory work?

Enter the spoon theory. Christine Miserandino came up with this idea when she used it to talk about how her lupus affected her ability to do everyday things.

Here's how it works: We all start with the same number of spoons in the morning, but every little task we do costs us a spoon. And some tasks require more spoons than others. Like going on a work trip—that'll drain your spoon supply faster than you buying too much at a Sephora sale. And don't even get me started on pain—it's like a spoon thief, stealing precious energy one spoonful at a time. So, if you take on too much, you'll end up with no spoons left in your kitchen drawer. So, you've got to be smart with how you use your spoons.

In the same way, your spoon count is based on how you live your life. Like how skipping a meal or not exercising takes away a spoon or two. Arguing with your health insurance company about coverage for a new prescription—say goodbye to two more spoons.

"Sorry, I can't. I have no spoons left."

Starting the day with ten shiny spoons is like winning the lottery. But when you wake up with stiff joints, it's like the spoon fairy came and snatched one away. And then you've got a meeting to rush to, so you sacrifice two more spoons just to shower and eat breakfast. And let's not forget about your furry friend who needs a walk—there goes another spoon. By the time you make it to work, 40 percent of your spoons are gone already.

Now, you've got to be really careful with those remaining spoons. If you use them up too fast, you'll be more drained and struggle throughout your work day. And you don't want to get stranded without any spoons left to make it home, do you? So choose wisely.

How to use it

The spoon theory isn't just helpful for you but for your loved ones too. You can easily tell your partner, "Babe, I've only got three spoons left," and they'll know to lend a helping hand. It's like having your own personal spoon squad. This theory will help you make better decisions and give you the power to do things that will make your life better. It will teach you how to conserve and restore your energy levels while being selective and intentional in your actions.

Planning your day is key. Need to give a big presentation? Prepare to use a lot of spoons, so don't waste them on trivial things like laundry or cooking dinner. Say no to activities that drain you and preserve your spoons for the most important tasks.

And don't forget the "firsts"—they can be a real spoon drainer. If you are injecting yourself with Benlysta for the first time or going to a new doctor, be prepared to use extra spoons. The good news is that self-care can replenish those spoons. Read a book, listen to your favorite music, play with your pet—basically, anything that brings you simple pleasure.

Remember, your spoon count and energy requirements will change based on your lupus levels, so adjust accordingly. Raise your spoons to the spoon theory and use your energy wisely.

Reflections

- Medical gaslighting is not okay. Stand up to that mo-fo.
- Get a second or third opinion if you think you are being misunderstood, ignored, or not taken seriously.
- Having lupus is a pain in the wallet, just saying.
- Use the spoon theory to strategically conserve energy throughout the day.

6

Be Your Own Bestie Advocate

My whole life changed when I realized I could be humble and calm yet still take no shit and set solid boundaries to protect my energy.

—Viola Davis

When I found out I had SLE, I was like, “Nah, not gonna tell a soul.” I had this whole superhero complex going on, thinking I had to be invincible no matter what. Showing any signs of weakness? No way, José. So, I kept it all hush-hush.

But then something shifted, and lupus became my get-out-of-jail-free card. I blamed it for everything under the sun, and I mean everything. “Don’t you dare give me plastic bags! Can’t you see I’ve got lupus?” It was my go-to excuse for anything and everything.

Deep down, I was actually scared that if I let people see what I was going through, they’d be like, “Meh, not my problem.” I worried my feelings would be as disposable as yesterday’s leftovers. So I decided to keep it to myself. Looking back now, though, I’m like, “Oops, my bad.”

I could’ve been a shining beacon of knowledge about a disease that most people didn’t even know existed. My experiences could have helped others going through the same stuff. But hey, back then, it was all about me and just trying to survive the lupus roller coaster. Now I understand the importance of advocacy, putting yourself first, and sharing the challenges you're going through.

You're not going to find anyone in this world who is going to treat you better than you. That's why this chapter is all about how to be your own bestie because you're grade-A amazing.

You'll learn about developing true self-care practices and finding the good in daily living. Last, we'll talk about how and why setting boundaries is important for staying healthy.

Self-Care

Ah, self-care, a broadly overused phrase in American culture, synonymous with filling up your own cup first. It is sold as a luxury, but it's a necessity when lupus is involved. It's about caring for yourself to make your mind, body, and spirit a nice place to live. It may be cliché, but it's for a good reason. Self-care is so important. Without it, your lupus could suffer more as you turn over your time and energy to people and things that aren't deserving of your awesomeness.

Real self-care cannot be bought. It's really not about a spa day with a sparkly unicorn bath bomb. It involves making tough decisions about what's best for you. It's choosing to be more disciplined, living in alignment with your values, prioritizing mental health, and putting your happiness front and center. Self-care is making the decision to remove toxic people from your life and selecting water over Diet Coke. "It's hard work, but not only can it be achieved, it can be maintained internally, unlike an off-the-shelf product or the lessons of a self-help guru," says Pooja Lakshmin, MD, author of *Real Self-Care*.

Sure, self-care can be selfish. You can and should put yourself first. When you do this, everyone around you benefits. How so? Because you become physically and mentally more available. Your cup is fuller, and you can draw more energy from it.

Self-care ends up being a band-aid if you settle for temporary solutions and don't address the underlying issues that bring on the stress, like taking a vacay from your crazy, chaotic job instead of working with your employer on a more manageable workload. Rather, learn to pick healthy behaviors and actions, like sleep and exercise, to replenish you and fill you up. These healthy things will help you deal with the real problem, calm you down, and keep you in the present.

There will be days when self-care means allowing yourself to feel anger, annoyance, and sadness. Go ahead: feel it, and let it pass. Working on calming down the mental chatter in your head, understanding your feelings, and choosing to replace negative thoughts with more realistic ones are acts of self-care. Plus, some days you won't care about doing "the work" on this, and there's no need to feel guilty about it. Everyone has these moments. Allow yourself to be human.

Self-Care Formula

Self-care is whatever the hell you want it to be as long as it (1) doesn't hurt anyone, (2) is legal in your state or country and (3) brings you joy. If it's working now, keep at it. Assuming, of course, that you aren't actually acting as a troll and being a total asshat to other people, which would be a violation of rule number one.

And self-care doesn't have to be extravagant or excessive. Small, simple actions are just as impactful, like a nice rest on your porch watching the sunset or eating a ripe peach as it drips down your face. Self-care is often synonymous with escaping or getting away from it all, but it can also mean stretching yourself and growing through experiences, like a guitar class.

Gratitude, Y'all

Think of the beautiful flowers in your yard, the kind stranger who held the door for you, or the police officer who let you go without a speeding ticket. This is gratitude at work here. It's focusing on what's good in our lives and being thankful for the things we have. Gratitude is pausing to notice and appreciate the things that we often take for granted, like having a place to live, food, clean water, and even wi-fi access.

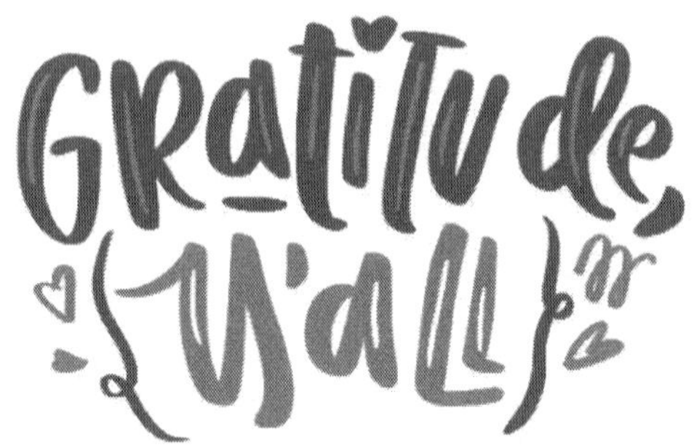

The cool thing about being grateful is that the more you pay attention to it, the more you see. It trains your brain to search for the good in life. If you change your point of view so that you are looking for beauty, excellence, and kindness, you can see more of those qualities around you. Indeed, tapping into feelings of appreciation has a profound impact on your mood, soul, and possibly your lupus.

It may sound crazy to try to find gratitude when you feel like a pile of poo, but it's worth it. **Even on the darkest of days, there's always something to be thankful for.** Maybe you woke up this morning with a roof over your head and some toilet paper to wipe your tushie. These little things are easily overlooked, but when they're gone, we realize just how much we miss them. Last winter, my house lost power for eleven hours, and let me tell you, when it finally came back on, I was over-the-moon grateful. And if you're really struggling to find something to be happy about, check out some lupus groups on Facebook or Reddit. Seeing others' deep lupus struggles will make you feel like you're almost normal.

"The key is to scan your environment regularly for things and people to appreciate rather than criticize. In doing so, you create a new climate of praise and gratitude in your life," says marriage expert and author John Gottman. Do this by creating a list of at least three things you're thankful for each day. It could be anything, big or small, like hearing birds sing or laughing at your bestie's joke. The more you practice, the easier it'll become to see the good in life. Keep that gratitude flowing, despite that asshole lupus getting in your way.

Keeping Yourself Mentally Healthy and Safe

Throughout your lupus quest, you've likely come across a variety of family, friends, and loved ones—some have lifted you up, and others have scorched you like a hot pan. You have a choice about what to put up with in your life and how people treat you. This is where boundaries come in. They help you stay healthy and safe while honoring your needs, much like fences between neighbors.

In *The Book of Boundaries*, author Melissa Urban says, "Boundaries are how we care, stay supportive, and give to those we love without sacrificing our own health and happiness in the process." They are about what you will and will not accept, and they involve making plans and choices about your life, like who and what you let in and what you keep out. Setting limits is vital for prioritizing your well-being, resolving conflicts, reducing stress, and helping to create a healthy sense of personal space.

You might need to set more boundaries if you find yourself:

- saying “yes” at your own expense
- feeling resentful and drained after interacting with that person
- being overrun and dominated in conversations and relationships
- tolerating others’ harmful behaviors out of fear of hurting feelings or retaliation

Boundaries are like a protective cloak; they prioritize your health and safety and sound a lot like:

- “I know what you want from me, but I will not be able to do this.”
- “We can agree to disagree on this. Let’s talk about something else.”
- “I need one hour of alone time after dinner.”
- “We will be celebrating Hanukkah at home. We will join you guys at 6 p.m.”

A boundary is really about your needs

Remember thinking that boundaries were just a way to boss people around and get them to change? Yeah, it turns out that’s not how it works. When you set boundaries, you’re not telling someone else what to do. You’re telling them what you will do if they don’t respect your desires and needs. And it’s not about changing them or making them “see the light.” It’s about taking care of yourself.

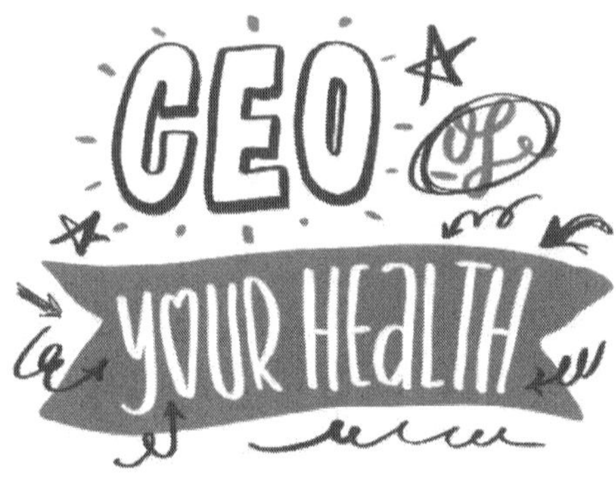

You don't have control over anyone else's actions, but you can control yourself, how you respond, and what you allow in your life. People don't need to change in order for you to feel satisfied and better. So, if your friend keeps sending you those lupus articles you don't want, you can just say "bye Felicia" and take a break from that friendship. And if your friend keeps you on the phone too long, you can politely end the convo. The point is, you've gotta protect yourself and what's important to you and set boundaries accordingly.

"Thanks, but I am not looking for feedback on my lupus care."

Let me tell you a personal story about the cost of a boundary that I set with my mother. For years, I kept quiet and allowed her to say and do hurtful things, fearing her reaction and thinking that speaking up would ruin our relationship. The relationship was eating away at my soul, and it was unhealthy for me at a time when I really needed my health to be a top priority.

But a few years later, when my daughter became involved, I knew I had to do something to protect her from experiencing the same pain and resentment that I did. After careful consideration, I made a difficult decision and laid down a limit with my mom to protect myself. Unfortunately, that was the end of our relationship (although I have hope that this will change one day). From this, I learned that I cannot control her or anyone else's actions. I am solely responsible for myself. As painful as it is to not have her in my life, I am okay with this because, mentally, I'm healthier and stronger.

"Daring to set boundaries is about having the courage to love ourselves even when we risk disappointing others," says Brené Brown. Setting boundaries can be 'effin hard for both you and the other person. It's not so easy to say no to something that you've put up with for thirty years from a loved one or to muster the courage to tell your boss that his comments were sexist and must stop. People fear that a boundary will result in a huge fight, bring on rejection, or end a relationship. That's a fair risk.

Others believe that their boundary-setting portrays them as mean or self-centered. Instead, they'd rather be kind and allow people to continue doing things that cause hurt and harbor resentment. Here's the kicker—what you don't address in your relationships, you ultimately approve. If you don't create a boundary to protect yourself, you're basically telling everyone else that they are more important than you. Is this what you really want?

How to set those boundaries

Now that you know why setting limits is good for you, your lupus, and your health, you might be wondering how to make your own.

Step 1: Identify the boundary you need at this time.

Find the boundary that is necessary for you right now, no matter if you've put up with it for decades or not. Lupus can put a damper on your energy levels, so it is important to think about what you really want and how realistic it is given your current situation. Determine what feels appropriate and healthy for you and what your non-negotiables are, like "I'm down for this but not for that." It's crucial to understand what you want from the relationship before establishing a boundary, since you can't control the other person, recommends author Nedra Glover Tawwab.

You can anticipate the other person throwing some guilt, blame, or judgment your way once you start setting your limits. This whole thing is new and will take some time to take effect.

Step 2: Set the boundary using "I" statements and in clear language.

Begin with statements like "I want," "I feel," "I need," and "I think." Taking personal responsibility for how you feel without blaming others reduces hostility and defensiveness from the get-go. Brené Brown taught us about boundaries when she said, "Clear is kind. Unclear is unkind." This means that no one can read your mind. Telling people what you think they want to hear is both unkind and fruitless. It also holds that person back from improving and can create bigger relationship problems in the future. Being clear about what you need and what you expect is best for boundary setting and in life.

Normalize telling people specifically what you need and want from them, or else you'll end up with a whole lot of crap you don't want or have space for.

A person doesn't have to agree with your boundary or even understand it in order to respect it. Also, you do not need to explain why you set a boundary. Just take a deep breath, state that boundary, and move on.

Step 3: Reinforce that limit.

Just because you set a limit once doesn't mean your work is done or that everyone will follow it right away. If you don't back up what you say, people learn not to listen to what you're requesting, and they'll push your boundaries aside while stepping on you in their pointy shoes. You may have to say the boundary again and again, perhaps in different ways, until it's finally honored.

Keep in mind that a boundary is not effective if there are no real consequences for breaking it. Outline the actions you are willing to take and allow for a gradual change. Your consequences do not have to be set in stone, but they do need to be firm. A consequence can sound like, "If you continue to give me advice on my lupus, I will ask you to leave."

Sometimes the smartest thing to do is to stay away from people who do not respect your limits.

Additional tips for better boundaries:

- Practice writing down your limits. This will make you more comfortable when speaking them out loud.
- Say nothing for ten seconds after setting a boundary. It's natural to want to fill the awkward silence with words, but don't back down from what you said.
- Have this conversation when you're alone with the person and the mood is calm.
- Never create a boundary that you can't or won't enforce.
- Don't apologize for setting a boundary.
- Keep in mind that it is equally important to respect others' boundaries.

Reflections

- Real self-care cannot be bought, and it takes hard work to put yourself first.
- Every day, think about all the good things that have happened to you.
- While a bit scary, setting boundaries is essential to your health and lupus.
- You cannot change what other people do, but you can change how you react and what you let into your life.

7
It's All About the Small Stuff

Sorry, there's no magic bullet. You gotta eat healthy and live healthy to be healthy and look healthy. End of story.

—Morgan Spurlock

One year after my diagnosis, I found myself in a mental rut. Despite diligently taking my medication, eliminating gluten from my diet, choosing walking over running, and plunging myself into knowledge about living with SLE, I felt like I wasn't making a real impact. It was as if all my efforts were in vain. The frustration was overwhelming, and I contemplated abandoning everything I had been doing. However, I took a moment of introspection and realized that beneath the surface, I was seething with rage. I was furious that I had done everything "right," and lupus was still able to come back. I had made sacrifices for the sake of my health, yet I still felt far from healthy. It hadn't fully sunk in that I couldn't control every aspect of my lupus.

Then a dose of reality hit me. Things could be far worse for me. Lupus could have wreaked even more havoc on my life, causing more damage to my internal organs and limiting my choices even further. As I shifted my perspective, I began telling myself, "I am grateful for the situation I'm in." Simply put, the healthier I was, the more manageable my lupus would be. Lupus has presented its own set of obstacles, but it hasn't taken away my ability to appreciate what I have. I choose to keep the majority of those healthy habits that are part of my daily routine and focus on the positive aspects that I have control over.

This chapter is all about finding ways to incorporate lasting, meaningful change that impacts your health and lupus. There's not one best way to do this, and small will ultimately make a big impact.

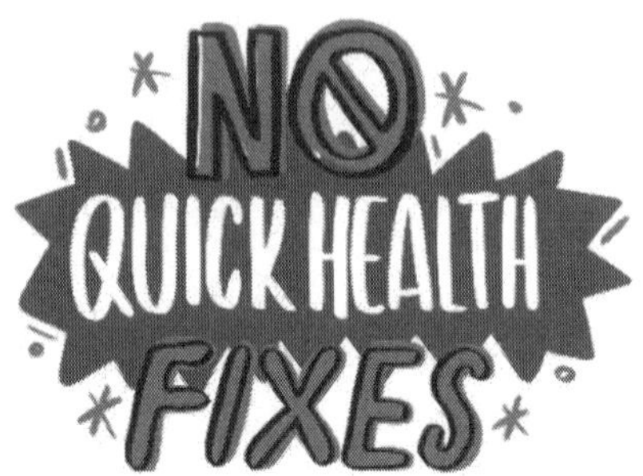

Daily Actions

Until a cure is found for lupus, managing the disease and its symptoms is the best way to maintain a good life. How you live and the decisions you make each day have a big impact on the quality of your life with lupus. "Many people don't connect how they feel to what they eat, how much they rest and sleep, how much they exercise, how much time they make for friends and community, as well as the media and news to which they expose themselves," says integrative physician Mark Hyman.

I'm not saying that prioritizing healthy habits and actions will make lupus disappear. You know better than that. There are no quick fixes to your health. But small changes done on repeat make teeny, tiny improvements in your health, like upgrading from an iPhone 11 to an iPhone 14. From here, you begin to stack these daily positive health actions, and you'll begin to feel better. Managing your lupus will be easier. And perhaps your life will begin to get a little bit better. Remember that you hold more power than your medical team because you get to control your thoughts, behaviors, and actions in life.

Little Things Matter

When we think about choices that have a big impact on our lives, we often think of big moments and actions, like climbing Mount Everest, becoming a vegan, starting your own business, or writing a best-seller.

In reality, the opposite holds true. It is the small, consistent actions we take every day that greatly influence our overall health. Simple things such as avoiding secondhand smoke, staying hydrated, and aiming for 6K steps daily yield larger, lasting, and positive results. By relying on these foundational habits, you can find stability amid the uncertainties of living with lupus.

These insights may seem obvious, which perhaps explains why we tend to procrastinate doing them. We continually put them off until a breaking point arrives, and we think, "Enough is enough. I can't continue like this anymore." Only then does change begin.

Ruled by habits

You are the sum of your habits—the things you do automatically. We make choices constantly throughout the day without even considering them. It's not just about routines; habits impact the way we eat, work patterns, and even our decision to take a walk or pour a glass of wine after a long day. Habits account for 40 percent of our behaviors. When this is combined with the fact that 47 percent of our lives are spent lost in thought, it's easy to slip into harmful patterns for our bodies, minds, and lupus.

Poor health choices accumulate— years of poor sleep, excessive drinking, and shitty eating habits take a toll. But here's the good news: Healthy choices also accumulate. Years of training, eating well, staying hydrated, and sleeping add up and protect you. The question is: How do you want to invest in yourself? Your future self will thank you for the actions you take today.

Creating meaningful health changes

Sometimes, good intentions aren't enough to bring about meaningful lifestyle or health changes. It's like wanting to start a support group for people lacking motivation but who just can't seem to find the energy to get it off the ground. Simply reading this book won't instantly revolutionize your approach to managing lupus. The key is to put in the effort to understand, adapt, and consistently practice these new skills until they become ingrained habits.

Change isn't easy and requires hard work. Wanting to change is just 5 percent of the equation. The remaining 95 percent is doing the work and creating healthy habits that will help you manage your lupus and be the type of person who does and lives the kind of kickass, amazing life she so desires.

Your daily actions hold immense importance, and you have control over them. Making changes in your habits requires setting goals with careful consideration for your thoughts and actions.

How to Create Healthier Habits

Connect to your "why"

Having a deep sense of purpose behind what you do in life makes it easier to adopt and maintain healthier habits. It acts as a guiding force, shaping your choices and behaviors. Your "why" gives you direction and a sense of purpose, which helps you stay focused even when things don't go as planned. Without it, you might feel lost or wander aimlessly, not knowing what you really want or what's truly important to you.

In the book *Atomic Habits*, James Clear talks about how we should first determine who we want to be and then act in that way. Starting with the question "Why is this important?" is the right move. Exactly what difference will this make in your life? You may want to be less stressed, but think deeper. Is it because you want to have a better work-life balance? Or would you like to have more time to work on a hobby like painting that brings you joy? Or take exercise. It can make you feel better about your body, but maybe your real reason is that you want to be able to get down on the floor to play with your grandson and then get back up again without help. Or you may want the energy and balance to climb up the bleachers to watch your favorite soccer team play.

Be aware that your sense of purpose will change as you go through life. This will lead you to find new ideas, passions, and paths.

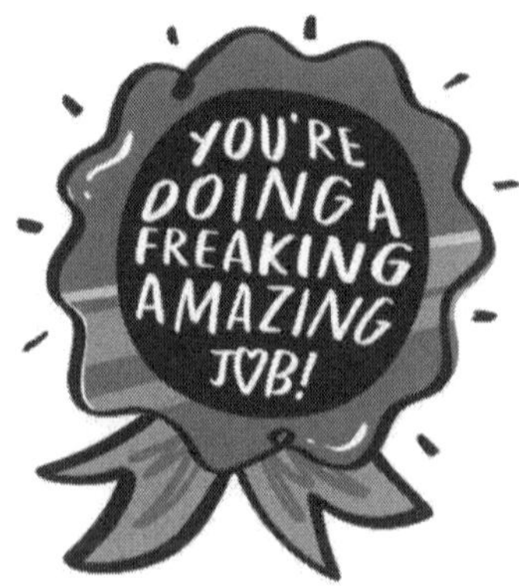

Small, realistic goals

If you want to form a habit that sticks, it's important to break it down into small, manageable bites. It's like breaking off a piece of chocolate instead of eating the whole damn thing. If your goal is too hard, you're more likely to toss it aside.

The more specific the goal, the better the chance of success, so get granular. For example, if the goal is to read more, ask yourself a bunch of questions to get down to the nitty gritty. Deciding: Why do you really want to read? What types of books do you like? How many pages do you want to read each day? How long do you want to read? Where and when will you do this? How will you track this action?

Make your desired habit so easy that you can stick to it even on the hardest of days. For example, you can practice deep breathing for one minute (versus setting a goal of meditating for fifteen minutes when you've never done a minute of it in your life) or limit your social media use to thirty minutes a day (versus being on Instagram for as long as you want).

A Word on Motivation

Relying solely on willpower to create a habit is the wrong approach. The most seemingly disciplined people in the world, like Rihanna and Serena Williams, lack motivation. Even these women don't have enough drive to get up and go every single day. This means that you've got to choose habits that you actually like and can keep up with. It's much harder to create a habit around something that requires a shitload of pump-up music to get you motivated to do it.

Be Consistent

The more you do something, the easier it gets to keep it going. With time, you can increase the duration and difficulty of the habit to make it more challenging. But it is important to put consistency ahead of intensity. Making small improvements over time is more likely to lead to long-term success than making a number of drastic changes all at once. If you put too much pressure on yourself too quickly, you may become overwhelmed and give up.

Exercise is one habit that can be difficult to start, especially if the gym is intimidating and you don't know where to begin. In this case, starting with tiny, achievable habits, like walking for five minutes a day, can be ideal. Then, over time, make the workout harder and longer, like walking on an incline for fifteen minutes.

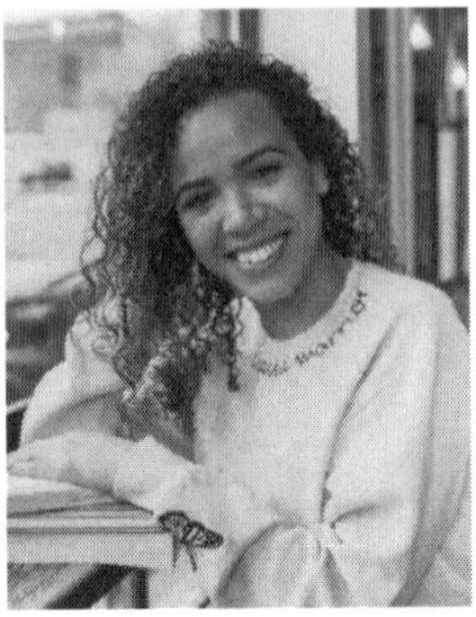

Lupus Warrior Profile

At @myloopylife, coach Selena Colon dedicates herself to guiding and empowering warrior women to forge their own paths toward thriving despite their lupus diagnosis. Selena's resounding message reverberates through the hearts of those she reaches: "Lupus isn't the end; it's a new beginning." Her words offer solace and the assurance that there is light at the end of the tunnel. Selena reminds women that there is hope and a brighter future ahead. She imparts the invaluable message that everything will ultimately fall into place. Selena's practical guidance on health underscores the importance of taking charge of one's well-being through lifestyle adjustments. Her influence stretches far beyond her coaching platform, leaving an indelible mark on those she guides with SLE toward a life of thriving and resilience.

Link to a positive

If you want to make a behavior a habit, connect it to a positive emotion right when you do it or immediately afterward. This way, you're more likely to remember it and keep doing it in the future. It's like giving yourself a little reward for taking positive actions, and it can make a big difference in forming healthier habits. Celebrate when you do what you said you were going to do, perhaps by dancing to your favorite song or by drawing a large red checkmark on your calendar and shouting, "Hell yeah!"

Routine connection

Developing a new habit can be hard, but one effective way to make it stick is by linking it with an already established habit or daily routine. With this, you can trick your brain into thinking the process is second nature. For instance, if you want to walk, you could decide to place your exercise clothes by your toothbrush. Keep an eye on your progress and make changes as needed. If you attempt a spot in your routine and it doesn't work, no worries. Just try another spot.

Track it

Did you know habit tracking is like motivation crack? Each small win becomes addictive, fueling your desire to keep going. Research shows tracking improves success rates for goals and makes them more likely to succeed compared to those who don't do this. Use a paper calendar, an app, or another method to mark your progress. That empty spot on the calendar becomes a powerful reminder not to break your streak and undo your hard work. There's an instant gratification in tracking—crossing off to-do list items or marking an X on a calendar. Why does it feel so satisfying? Moreover, tracking keeps you honest because it's either a yes or no; you can't deceive yourself. Focus on the process and be a person who does what she says she's going to do.

Enlist help

It's easy to let your health goals fall by the wayside when lupus dominates. That's why having a supportive friend check in can help you stay accountable. It's like having a personal trainer, therapist, and mom all rolled into one. When you try a shortcut or skip a workout, she's there to give you the side-eye and call out your BS. You may grumble and complain when she suggests the fruit over the glazed donut, but deep down, you know she's doing it because she cares about your health and well-being.

Be a Wary Chick: Don't Trust All You Consume

Are you afraid of using the wrong deodorant, worried about toxic chemicals in tampons, or scared of non-organic strawberries? The health and wellness industry, news outlets, and influencers are to blame for these fears. They use guilt and shame to make you feel like you are not good enough while promoting their products as the answer to being bright, happy, healthy, and cool. Author Rina Raphael, in *The Gospel of Wellness*, highlights how wellness convinces us that we can buy our way to better health.

Women play a significant role in healthcare decision making, accounting for 85 percent of all consumer purchases. We easily fall for health fads, and marketing companies are well aware of this, targeting our insecurities with their persuasive words and images. They employ the age-old method of making women feel bad about themselves to sell their products.

Science is constantly evolving too. Remember when smoking on airplanes was considered safe? Trust science to a certain extent, but always think critically and maintain skepticism about the information that influences your health.

Biotin is the perfect example for me. I was taking this supplement to help with my nails, which break so easily since starting Plaquenil. Biotin makes a big difference, but I stopped taking it after watching a physician on TikTok say it could hurt my thyroid. I don't even know what type of physician he is, yet I accepted what he said as factual. My nails became brittle again. I pondered why in the hell I trusted him and finally went back on biotin. My nails are fierce again. Go figure.

Don't trust everything you read or watch about your health, even if it's from a fellow lady with lupus. What works for her might not be the best for you.

You, my friend, are going to be wiser. No longer will you blindly accept what your feed and search engine offer you. Instead, you'll rely on reputable sources for your health. When you come across a claim, like how probiotics are great for lupus, you'll dig deeper before accepting it. The brilliant and formidable female scientists behind the Unbiased Science podcast offer valuable tips for evaluating online health advice:

1. Do they make claims that go beyond what they know?

2. Are they going against the advice of professionals or official medical bodies?
3. Do they recommend a cure, diet, or treatment that is not possible?
4. Do they make unproven claims about how safe their products are?
5. Do they rely on one study or a story instead of looking at the larger body of research?

If the answers to any of these questions raise concerns, it's time to find a more reliable source of information.

Reflections

- The daily routines you follow greatly determine your health.
- Change isn't easy or quick, but consistent actions win the race.
- For healthier habits, set small goals, link them to what you're already doing, and reward yourself when you reach them.
- Keeping track of your progress and asking a friend to hold you accountable helps a lot.

8

Squad Goals: Building Your Ultimate Support Posse

Ask for help, not because you are weak.
But because you want to remain strong.

—Les Brown

Sure, having lupus sucks, and having a daughter with lupus? Double the suckage. Once upon a time, I roamed as a lone lupus warrior, feeling like a zebra in a herd of horses. It was tough, no doubt about it. Not having anyone who truly understood the ups and downs of living with lupus left me feeling isolated and disconnected. I wanted someone to understand my constant tiredness, my unpredictable flares, and how hard it was to find my way through the medical maze.

But then Ahnna, my daughter, was diagnosed with lupus, and everything changed. Suddenly, I had an instant lupus bestie. Oh, what a difference it made! We formed a tight-knit tribe that understood the unspoken language of chronic illness and exchanged cuss words when the pain became unbearable. I felt safe in the knowledge that we were never truly alone in our fight. We had each other going forward. While this is a burden that I never wanted my daughter to bear, I am grateful to be able to provide her support and receive some in return. Our mother-daughter lupus bond makes even the darkest days feel a bit lighter and my future brighter.

This chapter is all about the different ways you can build a strong support system around your lupus diagnosis. We will talk about where to look for allies outside of your immediate circle and why it is totally fine to ask for help when you need it.

Sharing Your Diagnosis

Living with lupus is hard on many levels, one of which is the large lack of understanding in our society about this chronic illness. It's enough to deal with this shitty disease, but having to defend ourselves in front of others is draining and disheartening. Having to "prove" that you're sick enough to get others' attention is just wrong. And when the truth about how you are doing is finally shared, it can come off as too pessimistic. Because people will only tolerate you feeling bad for a set amount of time before they want to talk about something "good" for once.

When you do share your lupus diagnosis, be prepared for a variety of responses from people. Some may offer genuine support, while others may crack jokes, like my dad laughing about his own knee hurting and how he must have lupus too. Just remember, you can't control how others respond, but you can control how you react. So don't expect them to be saviors, because, let's be real, we're the ones fighting the damn lupus here.

Here are some of the most common things people say when you tell them you have lupus and the snarkiest ways to respond.

Stupid Comment: At least you don't have _____ (insert some other shitty ass disease like ALS or bulging eye syndrome).

Witty Response: Thank you for pointing out the fact that you don't feel I am sick enough to deserve your care and attention. I'll just remove you from my support list.

Stupid Comment: God never gives us more than we can handle.

Witty Response: This implies that God thinks I'm weak if I can't handle it. Plus, lots of other people can't handle what they get in life, so why force this crap on me?

Stupid Comment: Girl, just keep positive!

Witty Responses: Fuck off. Is that positive enough for you?

Stupid Comment: Have you tried yoga, paleo, or CBD?

Witty Response: Have you tried minding your own business? That works well too.

Continue to Share

When I share my lupus diagnosis, the most common response I get is "Isn't that what Selena Gomez has?" While it can be tiresome to repeatedly explain my illness, it remains crucial to do so. By increasing awareness and understanding, we shed light on the realities faced by those with SLE. This, in turn, paves the way for improvements in care and quality of life for individuals battling this disease and helps get the research fund greatly needed.

However, not everyone in your life needs to be privy to the details of your lupus journey. Sure, your loved ones genuinely care, but what about those nosy individuals and casual acquaintances? It's time to shut them out. Frankly, you don't have the energy to spare for their confusion and needless worry. With acquaintances, it's perfectly acceptable to reply with a simple "I'm fine," even when that couldn't be further from the truth. Does the mail carrier really need to know your current health status while delivering letters? Here's a thought: save your energy and share how you're really doing with someone truly deserving and trustworthy.

Choose to allocate your limited resources wisely, reserving them for the people and activities that truly matter. Surround yourself with those who uplift and support you, while sparing yourself the energy-draining burden of explaining your condition to those who don't matter. **Your well-being is precious, and you have the power to determine how it is shared and where it is best invested.**

Support Needed

In the face of lupus, your close friends and family become your personal squad of health superheroes. With their love, compassion, and support, your team becomes your ultimate ally, providing hope, laughter, and resilience as you navigate the absurd complexities of life with a chronic disease. Honestly, without them, life would be much harder. They listen without unleashing judgment, swoop in with comfort during moments of despair, and throw epic parties to celebrate the tiniest wins with an enthusiasm that could rival a victory parade. Their presence makes up for the fact that illness is unpredictable and reminds you that you are not fighting your condition alone.

"Get your shit together"
SAYS YOUR FRIEND WHO CLEARLY DOESN'T HAVE HERS FIGURED OUT

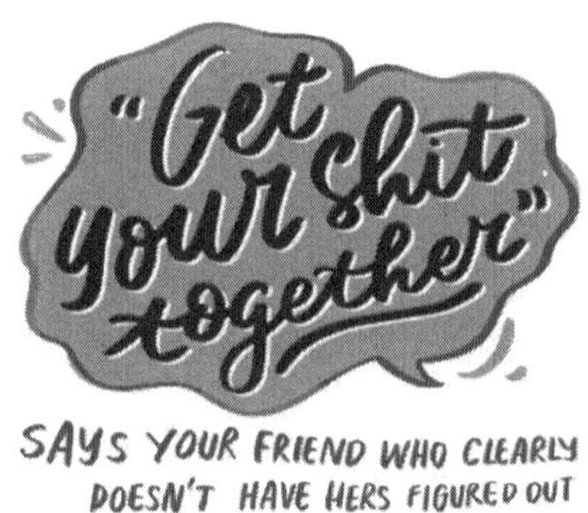

Pick and Choose

To ensure your own well-being as a lupus rockstar, it's crucial to have the right people around. The truth is, you must be selective about the people you allow into your life, as your relationships directly impact your well-being.

Take the time to determine if someone is the right fit for you. Are they deserving of your valuable energy and time? Is there mutual give and take? Do they genuinely care about your health and well-being? Is there excessive drama surrounding them?

Keep the cherished mix of family members and friends who uplift and fill you with joy and positivity. For the people who drain your energy, it's essential to distance yourself from them.

However, don't hesitate to end an established relationship if it's bringing you down or no longer feels fulfilling. Whether it's a friend from sixth grade or your cousin you grew up peeing in the kiddie pool with, you have permission to let go of unhealthy or toxic connections. Your well-being should always take precedence.

This also means to shun or remove those people that make you experience FOMO or make you feel inadequate just by watching them, both in your personal life and on social media.

Create a Support Caucus

Are you tired of having to repeatedly explain your lupus diagnosis to family and loved ones? Wish there was a way to streamline the process and ensure everyone understands and supports you? Well, fret no more! Allow me to introduce you to the concept of a "support caucus"—a term borrowed from the world of government but adapted to suit your lupus journey.

Gather your trusted core tribe for a special meeting. This is where the magic happens. Share with them the ins and outs of your SLE diagnosis, providing them with all the important details you've gathered thus far. Paint a vivid picture of what living with this disease entails—the unpredictability, the twists and turns, and the constant adjustments it demands. Be open and transparent about your needs, both in the present and the future. And don't forget to give your tribe the floor to ask questions, express their fears, and voice their concerns.

Within this support caucus, you can tackle a range of topics. From discussing how to approach the topic of lupus with your children to devising the best strategies for upcoming medical appointments, no stone should be left unturned. Your tribe can even brainstorm ways to handle inquiries from nosy neighbors or curious acquaintances. For instance, when the pushy neighbor says, "Hey, I heard Tanisha is sick with lupus," your support caucus can politely tell her to butt out by responding: "It's complicated, and Tanisha can share more when she's ready."

By establishing a support caucus, you create a united front—a team of individuals who not only understand your condition but also stand by your side. Together, you can navigate the challenges of lupus, find comfort in shared experiences, and empower each other to face the world with confidence. Remember, you deserve a network of unwavering support, and the support caucus is your ticket to ensuring everyone is on board with your lupus quest.

Like-Minded Support

When it comes to dealing with lupus, sometimes your friends and family don't have the bandwidth or time to help and provide support. That's why it can be a lifesaver to surround yourself with other like-minded lupus warriors. These women can truly understand what you're going through because they too are on their own journey. It's like a little tribe of fellow sufferers who can commiserate and share their coping strategies. And let's be real, sometimes it just feels good to vent to someone who truly gets it. You can find others who understand what it is like to live with lupus through social media, support groups, and professional lupus assistance.

Social Media

The power of social media has expanded far beyond the simple act of sharing photos and is now being used to forge strong bonds of friendship, like those between women who share the hardships of SLE. There is no denying that, when used with caution and moderation, social media provides a valuable source of friendship without ever having to leave the comfort of your phone. For me, many of my lupus friends were found on Instagram. This platform can help people get to know each other, make friends, and accept each other by giving comfort, support, and a sense of belonging outside of the virtual world.

While platforms like Facebook and Reddit serve as go to social media forums, it's important to remember that these peer-to-peer health groups should not replace medical advice. While they have some guidelines and a moderator to keep things in check, sometimes things can slip through the cracks. Go ahead and connect with your lupus tribe, but don't forget that your physician knows best.

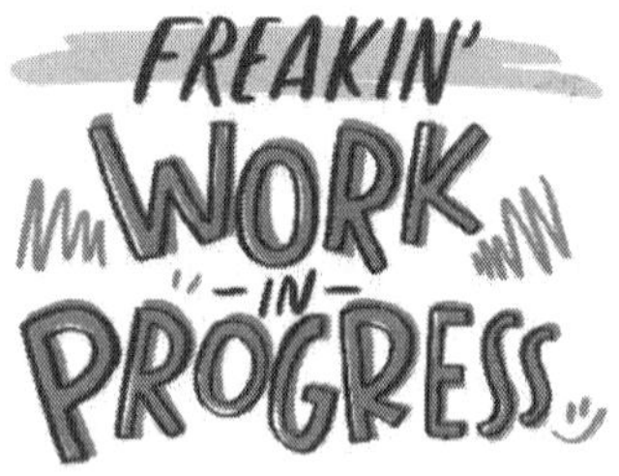

Support Groups

Whether it's in-person or online, support groups have become a vibrant space for lupus warriors to connect, discuss burning questions, and receive support from fellow community members who understand their experiences. They also remind you that you're not alone in this chronic disease battle. And hey, thanks to the pandemic, virtual meetings online are more popular than ever, offering a flexible way to connect from the comfort of your own home to get nurtured and supported while being less isolated.

A bonus is that these groups are often free. For help finding these, check out local hospitals or mental health centers for local offerings on lupus, autoimmune diseases, and/or pain management. You can also find a variety of groups offered at one of the nonprofits below.

Outside Support

There are some great nationwide nonprofit support resources available for you to get additional help with managing your lupus. Here are my top three recommendations:

The **Lupus Foundation of America** (LFA) funds studies and fellowships and provides resources to those needing guidance. They offer over 108 different support groups, including those tailored to specific demographics (Asians, Hispanics, caregivers, and so on). There are also local state chapters that provide community resources. I've used them to find a rheumatologist in NC and a local support group in my area. You can also go with LFA to Washington, DC, to advocate for equitable access to lupus care with your representatives in Congress, like I did in 2023.

Kaleidoscope Fighting Lupus is a global organization that serves as a hub for the lupus community, scientists, and medical professionals. Their focus is on fostering a supportive network and raising awareness about this disease. Kaleidoscope offers emergency financial assistance, on-the-ground support groups, and advocacy efforts to provide immediate and long-term help for those with lupus.

The **Lupus Research Alliance's** (LRA) ultimate goal is to revolutionize the way lupus is treated and cured. To achieve this, LRA is committed to funding cutting edge lupus research, supporting a diverse pool of scientific talent, promoting collaboration between researchers, and striving toward better diagnostics and more effective treatments. What they can offer you is education, access to resources, and an online community where you can give and receive support.

Asking for Help

Many of us find ourselves in the role of being reliable support systems for others. However, it's interesting to note that we often struggle when it comes to receiving help and supporting ourselves. We have a hard time asking for or accepting assistance, even from those who genuinely love and care about us. It's our fear of vulnerability and judgment that often prevents us from seeking support and opening up, leading us to believe we can handle everything on our own. However, refusing to ask for help only adds unnecessary stress and pressure to our already inflamed lives. **We all need someone to lean on at times, and you are no exception.**

Here's the thing: People who know and care for you would be tickled pink if you asked them to do something for you because they would love nothing more than to see you happy and healthy-ish. Being your trusty sidekick makes them feel all tingly inside and shows that you trust and have confidence in their skills. Asking for help is a good thing, not a sign of weakness. You don't always have to be the one who has it all together.

This leads to the specifics of how to ask for help. If at all possible, begin a discussion when you're feeling good and your pain is low. Make a list of two to four people you could ask for favors from. Have a conversation with them about how lupus gets the best of you at times and tell them that you may need their help in the future. Give some examples of the type of support needed, and ask if and how they are willing to help out. Don't wait until things become dire for you and it becomes an emergency before finding assistance.

Reflections

- Be a picky chick and carefully choose who will be on your support team.
- Find comfort in connecting with other warriors who understand your SLE experience, either online or on social media.
- Explore lupus-focused nonprofit support groups across the country to find more ways to deal with your condition.
- Asking for assistance is not a sign of weakness, and those who care about you would be delighted to help out.

9

Sidekicks and Superheroes: The Power of a Support Team

To be fully seen by somebody, then, and be loved anyhow—this is a human offering that can border on miraculous.

—Elizabeth Gilbert

The week of April 10, 2023, was tough for me due to tight deadlines, extra stress, and, oh yeah, lupus being an asshole again. It was a slow buildup to a looming flare. On Wednesday that week, the totality of it all hit me, and I emotionally collapsed, shifting into a survival mode that involved a lot of tears. I flat-out refused to talk to my husband, Noi, a first for me. He was out of town, which made this easier. You see, I just could not stomach hearing another "It will be all right" pep talk from him. I felt like he had nothing to add that could ease my suffering, and I was equally sad and annoyed by this. On Noi's end, this request was easily honored, and he figured I would talk when I was ready. But I was flabbergasted. "How is he okay with this? Doesn't he want to be all supportive and lovey-dovey when I feel like shit? Where's the disconnect?" I wondered.

Lucky for me, the things I learned while writing this book helped me a lot. I came to realize that it was perfectly acceptable for me to seek solace in isolation as a means of self-preservation. Despite being married for twenty-three years, he still couldn't read my mind—thankfully, that is! That meant I needed to collect my thoughts and help him help me. I also knew the importance of talking to Noi about how to best support me during hard times and what I needed from him going forward.

Get ready for some relationship connections in this chapter. We'll examine how your family, friends, and trusty sidekicks can support you through lupus. Discover the genius of a ranking system that effortlessly explains your lupus status, and brace yourself for the vital role girlfriends play in this chaotic journey.

Your Support Clan

Relationships require energy and a committed investment to grow. When this happens, your relationship has a better chance of flourishing, and it fills you up. Makes sense. But what happens when you don't have the necessary elements to invest because lupus has robbed you of them? At times, it's either your health or your relationship, and you can only choose one.

Don't get a chronic illness. It's very inconvenient for others.

It's common for women to feel alone and misunderstood in their relationships with regards to SLE. There is also the added pressure of feeling like a burden. Even if you know your partner cares and wants to help, you may still feel bad about their extra housework or canceling plans because you're not feeling well.

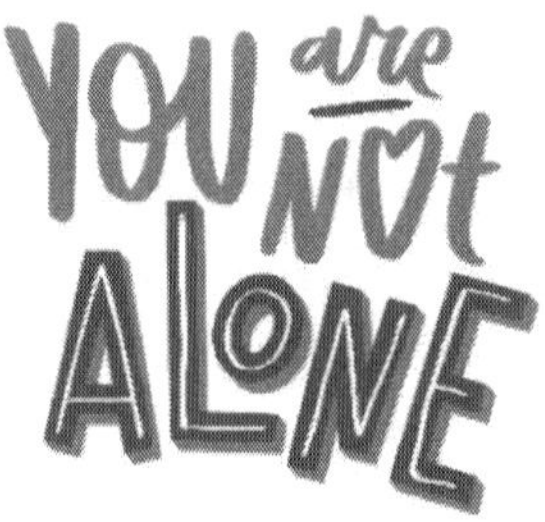

How to Help

First things first, encourage your partner to join you on your lupus quest as a couple. Invite them to learn everything they can about lupus. Remind them not to be afraid to ask you questions, but make sure they know not to offer any lupus advice. Going to rheumatology appointments or discussing blood work together can be another way for them to show their support. Then, they can work on upping their empathy game—it'll come in handy in all walks of life. Keep in mind that both you and your partner have the right to ask for some space in order to deal with the stresses brought on by SLE. It is a lot to think about and deal with.

While it's fair to be patient with your partner as adjustments are made to this new disease, it's not helpful if they remain stuck in denial or are continuously unsupportive. You totally know that you don't have to suffer through anyone invalidating your feelings, right?

Use a Ranking System

When I was in a flare, it was too taxing to tell my husband how I was doing over and over each day. It was yet more proof that I wasn't well. So together, we created a ten-point ranking system that made it easier for me to be honest with him. When he asked, "How are you today?" I could respond with a number and share where my lupus was without much effort. He then knew how to best respond to and care for me.

When you don't want to get into the nitty-gritty with your loved one, consider using a ranking system. Here's a breakdown of what each number means for us:

1. I feel good. Hey, want to go on a hike this weekend?
2. Pain is very minimal. Press on.
3. I could be better, so I hope this passes soon.
4. Hmm, this pain is hurting.
5. Keep an eye on me. I'm not feeling so well.
6. Pain is a constant. Stay close and offer support.
7. I'm bad! Get out my flare plan.
8. Stay home from work or have someone check on me.
9. Pain dominates my mind and body. I need you close by constantly.
10. Warning! Take me to my doctor or the ER, stat.

Female Friends

"Social support is the biggest factor that can positively affect happiness," says author Ruth Whippman in her book *The Pursuit of Happiness*. Friends who have your back and are willing to give and take are the best kind. And you don't need a big team; having just one or two allies in your corner can be enough. "Strong bonds are a female superpower," says Rina Raphael in *The Gospel of Wellness*. Research shows that close female friendships are more important for women than they are for men. Female friendships offer escape, relief, and refuge. And during times of stress, friends can provide a much-needed buffer.

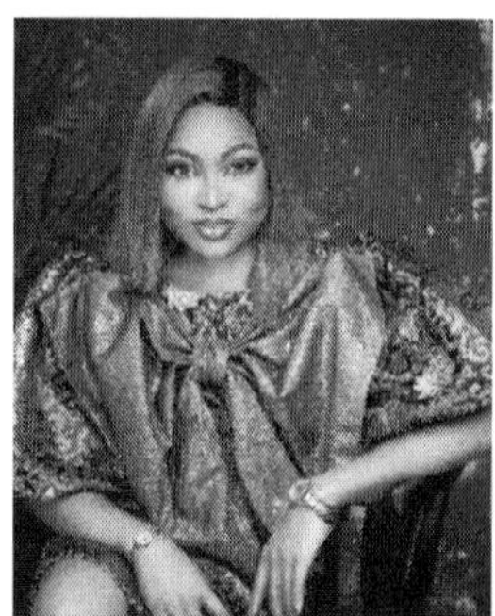

Lupus Warrior Profile

Precious Otiora (@previous_oti) stands as a beacon of inspiration with her empowering motto: "Lupus doesn't have me. I'm going to beat lupus!" Her resilience shined through as she established an online community that serves as a haven for lupus thrivers, fostering support and a sense of camaraderie. Precious's guidance for those grappling with a recent diagnosis is invaluable. She stresses the significance of conducting extensive research to bolster one's awareness of SLE while maintaining a vigilant eye on one's symptoms. Understanding the pivotal role of a strong support system, Precious emphasizes the necessity of surrounding oneself with people who contribute to a healthy network. Establishing personal boundaries and honoring the boundaries of others are crucial aspects of this process. With her compassionate yet assertive voice, she encourages women to discern and filter advice, focusing only on what is positive and genuinely beneficial for their own unique quest.

Give this book to your boo, bestie, mom, or auntie to read the paragraphs below. You can thank them later.

For the Friends and Support Team

Even if you don't know what to say or do, there are ways you can still be a great support system for that lovely woman of yours that has lupus.

What to Say

The woman you truly care about wants you to provide support and guidance no matter what comes her way, but you may be uncertain how to do this because you're afraid of saying the wrong thing. To begin with, the easiest thing to say is a heartfelt "I'm sorry to hear this" when the diagnosis is shared. It conveys concern and care all at once. Other suggestions that feel like a warm hug include:

- Thank you for sharing what's going on with you.
- I'm here for you.
- Take your time. I'll be here when you are ready.
- You have a beautiful heart; lupus can't touch this.
- How can I best support you?
- Tell me more about lupus and how it affects you.
- I love spending time with you, even when you're not okay.

When in doubt, be honest and ask her for guidance: "I don't know what to say. This is all new to me. How can I help you?" If you say something stupid or wrong along the way, it's okay. We all make mistakes. Sincerely apologize, and do better next time.

Learn everything you can about lupus so you're not completely lost. And don't be afraid to ask questions. Seriously, ask away. But be prepared for some unpredictable answers because lupus is like a box of chocolates: you never know what you're gonna get.

A phone call or text message can go a long way toward showing care and concern. It can sound like this, "How are you doing today?" Or "Do you want to share what's going on with you now?" But also know that words aren't the only way to show you care. Silence is also golden, and you can sit on a couch together while holding hands.

Even if she does not ask, doing things like getting her dinner, running errands, or getting her mail can go a long way. Be open to changing your plans based on how she feels. Instead of going out to dinner, plan to stay in, have a pajama party, and maybe watch a movie. You are still able to spend time with the person who is most precious to you. Remember, if your loved one is pushing you away when she's feeling bad, it's nothing personal.

Nope, Don't Say This

Let's move on to what not to say to a loved one who is sharing her lupus diagnosis or challenges.

To begin with, **don't offer up shallow, toxic positivity**. In hard times, no one wants to be told to "look on the bright side." While these comments are meant to be well intentioned and sympathetic, they come off as alienating and callous. I get it —looking at the positives makes you feel better. You hope that your loved one with lupus will have faith that the big, bad, and impossible challenges we're facing are actually making us stronger. But she just wants to know you are on her side. Even if you can't help her feel better, you can always help her feel seen. "The best way to support her is not by cheering her up but rather by showing up," reminds author Adam Grant.

PLEASE LET ME
KARATE CHOP
THE NEXT PERSON
WHO TELLS YOU
EVERYTHING HAPPENS
FOR A REASON
(Totally sorry you're going through this)

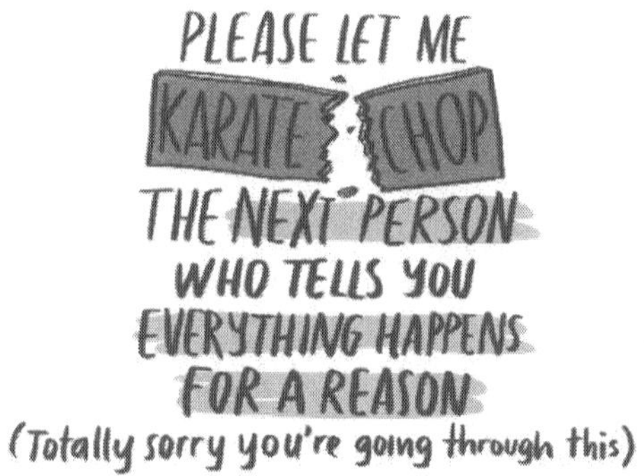

Avoid saying phrases like "I know how you feel," since it can come across as dismissive. Additionally, **please don't bloody give her advice!** Real love is simply being there. While you may feel uncomfortable, let your loved one share her feelings without needing to fix her. Meet her where she's at. It's her quest to go through, not yours to rescue her on.

More Empathy Please

When it comes to expressing care, support, and love, empathy is far more effective than sympathy. Let's talk about the difference, because there's a big one. Empathy feels how you feel. Sympathy hears how you feel.

Empathy thinks, "I don't know what it's like to have lupus, but I can relate to feeling scared. You're not alone." It's the willingness to try to understand what she's going through by connecting it to some similar experience you've had in the past. With this view, you're more relatable.

Sympathy, on the other hand, says, "Hmm, that lupus stuff sounds really bad. So, what do you want for dinner?" It's offering up sorrow for someone else's suffering or experience. And who wants someone's pity? This tends to make people feel alone and more isolated.

Turn to empathy as often as you can. It builds connection, over and above the words offered, and creates a bridge between you and your loved one with SLE.

Listen Better

The best thing you can do to support someone with lupus is to just listen. In a world filled with constant distractions, truly listening can be challenging. Our instinct is to offer solutions or change their perspective, but what matters most to women with lupus is being heard without judgment. To show you care, practice the art of silence and genuinely listen to her side of the story.

It's important to acknowledge that you can't solve her lupus problem or fully comprehend her experience. Instead, ask better questions that show comfort and compassion. For instance, a simple question like "How are you doing today?" acknowledges the difficulties of living with lupus and focuses on the present moment. Pepper your conversations with phrases like "Do you want to talk about it?" or "I love you. I care about you." Lastly, the question "Do you want to brainstorm on ideas, or do you want me to just listen?" points out a choice between your loved one's desire to be heard and wanting to hear some of your suggestions.

The simple way to show you care is to seal those lips, shut up, and listen to learn.

What matters most to women with lupus is being heard without judgment. To improve your listening skills, minimize distractions and maintain eye contact when she speaks. If you are distracted when she wants to talk, ask her for a raincheck. Approach the conversation with curiosity, and resist the urge to interrupt or provide immediate feedback. Let her finish talking before you answer. Put what you heard into your own words and ask for clarification if necessary; for example, "You're furious that lupus crushed your dreams of becoming a WWE wrestler, but you hate getting sweaty. Did I get that right?"

Remember that you cannot control her actions or decisions, even if you wish to. It can be frustrating when she doesn't meet your expectations, but ultimately, you have no control over her choices.

Lastly, remember that it's not about you. Your partner's actions are not meant to hurt you or the relationship. She is doing her best, and she would greatly appreciate your ongoing care and support as both of you navigate this disease together. Thank you very much.

Now give this book back to your beloved lady with lupus.

Reflections

- When dealing with lupus, the support of loved ones is crucial.
- You can keep your cool and give your pain a number with the help of a ranking system.
- Your team of cheerleaders has learned not only what to say to you but also what not to say.
- With more empathy and better listening skills, they can connect with you on a deeper level.

10

Your Beautiful Brain on Lupus

Your happiness is not contingent on someone else's understanding of you.
—Kiran Devaraj, MD

My first visit to a neurologist was a moment I had built up in my mind to be the answer to all my problems. I was so ready to uncover the issues behind my brain zaps—those electrifying sensations that had turned my head into a cosmic light show. Little did I know that the neurologist's response would be as unremarkable as a wet noodle.

When I poured out my heart and described my brain confusion, memory issues, and dizziness, I expected the neurologist to be concerned, or at least perplexed, by what was going on. But alas, what followed was an underwhelming response.

The neurologist, seemingly unimpressed by the celestial fireworks happening in my brain, simply ordered a scan. I thought, "Ah, finally! The moment of truth!" As I lay inside the MRI, my mind raced with visions of groundbreaking discoveries—tiny neurons dressed in lab coats, analyzing my brain zaps with furrowed brows. But when the results came in, the neurologist's verdict was a resounding "Okay." Apparently, my brain appeared normal to his well-trained eyes.

I couldn't help but chuckle at the absurdity of it all. Here I was, hoping for a eureka moment—a finding that would change my brain for the better. Instead, I got a "meh" that echoed through the halls of my neurologist's office. But hey, this is just another example of my test results appearing normal while my body said otherwise.

Let's talk about how lupus can really mess with your brain in a pretty unique way. Anything that affects the brain is pretty darn scary, right? Your first instinct might be to just ignore these symptoms and hope they magically disappear. But guess what? That's not going to help you in the long run. You'll need to know what's normal when lupus impacts your brain and when you should get help. This is what you'll find in this chapter, along with information on neuropsychiatric lupus and brain fog and how to cope.

Neuropsychiatric Lupus

Complications of the nervous system are some of the most common issues experienced with lupus and can show up as tingling, seizures, confusion, memory issues, headaches, dizziness, and much more. Inflammation often attacks the delicate structures of the nervous system, so these SLE problems persist. However, knowing this doesn't make them any easier to deal with.

There's a special kind of lupus that attacks your brain and nervous system called neuropsychiatric lupus (NPSLE). NPSLE is the least understood manifestation of lupus and affects 50 to 90 percent of those with SLE.[21 22] It's a scary problem that causes significant issues.

But first, a little science refresher: Your body is like a well-oiled machine, and the central nervous system (CNS) and peripheral nervous system (PNS) are like the mechanics that keep it running smoothly.

The CNS is like the control center of your body—it includes your brain and spinal cord, which work together to process and coordinate all the information that comes in from your senses and send out commands to the rest of your body. It's like having a personal assistant who's always on top of things, making sure everything runs smoothly. This extremely complex system is responsible for your hatred of raw onions, your love of the smell of fresh-cut grass, the regulation of your blood pressure, and your ability to do a sweet-ass version of the Electric Slide at weddings.

Now the PNS includes all the nerves that branch out from the CNS and extend throughout your body, kind of like a bunch of messengers running around and dropping off important notes. The PNS is divided into two parts—the somatic nervous system, which controls voluntary movements like talking or dancing, and the autonomic nervous system, which controls involuntary processes like digestion and sweating.

The CNS and PNS work together like peanut butter and jelly to keep your body running smoothly. Until that shitty lupus enters, then they don't get along so well.

How NPSLE Shows Up

Neuropsychiatric lupus can cause a variety of symptoms, such as forgetfulness, confusion, and mood swings. Imagine your brain throwing a party, but instead of good music and tasty snacks, it's serving up attacks and hallucinations. Yeah, it's not a party you want to attend. NPSLE can be minor, like "Eek, I'm forgetful today," all the way to "OMG, it feels like I'm having a stroke." My daughter and I have similar NPSLE experiences, which we call our "brain zaps." This is where we get random, sharp, shooting pains in our brains that cannot be explained any other way. It usually shows up during a flare and makes us freak the hell out.

The most common ways neuropsychiatric lupus shows itself include:

- cognitive dysfunction
- headaches
- peripheral issues (burning, tingling, or numbness)
- psychiatric conditions (depression or anxiety)
- memory loss (Huh? I've forgotten what you said already)
- seizures
- strokes, aneurysms, and transient ischemic attacks (pre-strokes)

Treatment and the Unknown

While the majority of the NPSLE concerns are short-lived and minor, they remain scary and overwhelming to deal with. There is no established cure for NPSLE. Management depends on the symptoms and the underlying causes. To me and everyone else who deals with NPSLE, this sucks ass.

It's a major downer that science is still trying to figure out exactly what causes NPSLE and how it affects the nervous system, but they think antibodies and inflammation may play a role.[23] [24] Can we please get on this, scientists? It remains a frustrating and challenging symptom of lupus that lacks the science to guide physicians and sufferers down a path toward help.

Often, you will be referred to a neurologist to diagnose and manage your NPSLE. That physician may be challenged to determine whether your neuropsychiatric symptoms are due to changes in your nervous system, stress from having a long-term illness, or some other factor. It's like trying to figure out if your mood swings are due to hormonal changes or just because you haven't had your morning coffee yet. And unfortunately, there is no specific test that can diagnose a neuropsychiatric complication of lupus.

In the meantime, this means your doctor has to use their own experience and recommendations, along with case studies and trial data, to figure out how to best help you. Treatment can include NSAIDs, steroids, and other symptomatic agents, like anti-seizure medications, for less threatening symptoms.

You can be proactive in the meantime and pay close attention to any new or existing mental symptoms that arise. Don't be afraid to speak up and share these changes with your doctor, no matter how weird or embarrassing they might seem. It's better to address them sooner rather than later, so you can get some sweet, sweet relief from the lupus fuckery that's messing with your brain.

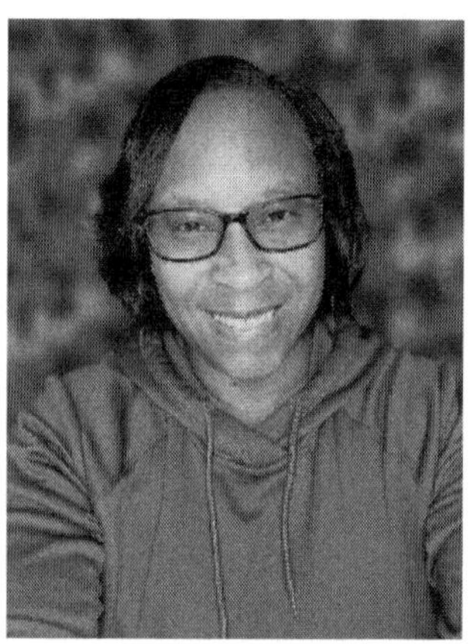

Lupus Warrior Profile

Racquel Dozier's impact as a lupus advocate and community builder is immeasurable. Her unwavering resilience in the face of multiple autoimmune conditions serves as an inspiration to others, while her transformative encounter in her younger days fuels her dedication to the positive mind-body connection at @LupusInColor. Racquel's selfless commitment to providing accessible resources, sharing personal experiences, and encouraging healthy habits resonates deeply within the community she has cultivated. Through her own quest, she instills hope, resilience, and self-advocacy skills, ultimately transforming the way individuals perceive and navigate their lupus diagnosis. Racquel's words, "**Give yourself some grace and compassion and don't compare your fight,**" are a powerful reminder to honor the body's limitations and exercise patience in understanding the complexities of one's diagnosis. With empowerment, Racquel guides women toward understanding, acceptance, and a renewed sense of internal strength.

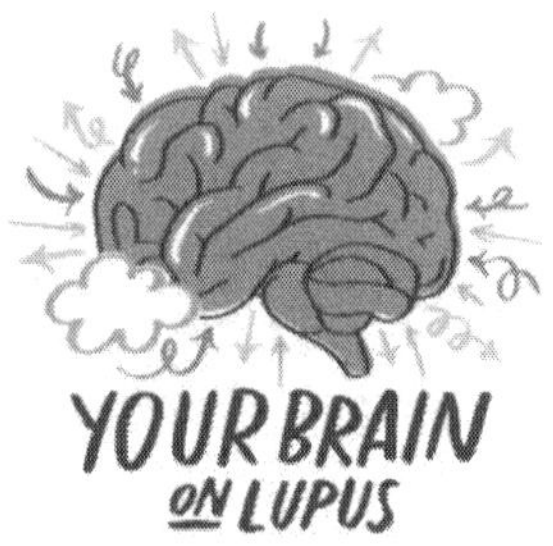

Brain Fog

Mental cloudiness and difficulty concentrating are symptoms of cognitive dysfunction, also known as brain fog. It is that feeling of your brain playing hide and seek with your ideas, and it seems like every thought is running late for a train that left the station ages ago. For me, it is like being stuck in a thick fog where everything is blurry and I am easily confused and forgetful.

While SLE brain fog can feel similar to the effects of profound stress or sleep deprivation, it's not the same. It is the most common SLE neurological condition, with up to 70 to 80 percent of people with SLE experiencing it at some point. This brain fog doesn't normally worsen over time, as it would with dementia or Alzheimer's disease. Memory problems, like other lupus symptoms, are likely to come and go, making life a bit more unpredictable. For some unlucky souls, brain fog can last for years and is sometimes worse for those who also have fibromyalgia.

While brain fog shows up differently in different people, some of its hallmarks include:

- inability to think clearly
- memory issues

- confusion
- trouble concentrating
- difficulty finding the right word
- needing to read things multiple times
- not being able to keep up with a conversation
- taking a long time to solve problems or make plans

Causes of Brain Fog

The exact cause of lupus brain fog is not completely understood (shocking, I know), but it is believed to be a result of inflammation in the brain as well as other factors.

Fatigue and stress can contribute and weaken the immune system. When your brain is exhausted, it is increasingly challenged to focus and process information.

Lack of sleep can interrupt how well your brain operates. Sleeping too little can lead to cloudy thoughts and poor engagement.

Certain **foods, sensitivities, vitamin deficiencies, and/or allergies** can all have a big impact on brain fog.

Inflammation can affect the blood vessels in the brain, leading to reduced blood flow and oxygen to the brain cells and resulting in cognitive impairment. In addition, lupus can also cause damage to the CNS, which contributes to brain fog.

Steroids and immunosuppressants, which are commonly used to treat flares, can worsen brain fog and also cause cognitive side effects like confusion, forgetfulness, and trouble focusing.

Coping with This Fogginess

First things first, talk to your rheumatologist if brain fog is putting a strain on your life. Typically, they'll need to figure out what's causing the problem before it can be fixed. There is no official way to test for brain fog, and people who have it may look completely healthy. So, doctors have often missed the condition or, worse, written it off. You may need to see a neurologist to change your medications or a counselor to learn new ways to cope with stress.

Just because brain fog is so common with SLE, this doesn't mean that you should just roll over and accept that the fogginess is there to stay.

Instead, there are methods that you can put to use that will lessen memory and concentration issues.

1. Plain and simple, **if you need help remembering things, do not rely on your brain for this**. Everything you need to remember, from appointments and tasks to passwords and the location of your spare set of car keys, should be written down. Making lists and notes jogs your memory and takes the burden of remembering off your shoulders. You can do this in a notebook or on your phone; just stick to the same method so that you don't find gibberish written on random scraps of paper. Check your notebook or device daily to make sure you're not missing anything.
2. Still feeling forgetful as shit? **Ask someone to remind you**. As in, "Hey, can you remind me to buy more tampons today?" Sure, the other person will probably forget to tell you this unless she has a topnotch memory. What this actually does is make your memory stronger because you said it out loud. It's also important to tell others if you have memory issues so they know what's going on and what to expect from you. This isn't an excuse; it's the truth.
3. Did you know that tidying up your home and workspace can help your mind feel more organized? Disorganization can bring on extra stress. Simply being in a cluttered room pulls your focus away from what you are working on and into the chaos around you. Brain fog can make you forgetful, and a lack of organization makes this worse. Being organized allows your brain to focus on what's necessary instead of being pulled into the realm of distraction. Your brain needs to be freed from as many intrusions as possible.

MULTITASKING bullshit

4. Institute a total ban on multitasking. I know you feel like you can chop some garlic while watching Gray's Anatomy. That's because your focus is really on the show and not the task. But try writing an email while listening to a friend tell you about the cute jump suit she scored on Poshmark—that's hard. Despite thinking that women are much better than men at this, the brain is not able to

split and complete two tasks at once. It's no good for the mind and accounts for a 10 percent drop in IQ, a 40 percent drop in productivity, and 50 percent more mistakes. When we think too much and try to do too many things at once, we miss out on life. Instead, adopt a mindset of monotasking—be diligent and only do one thing at a time. Turn off your phone and email when you really need to get work done. You might also find it helpful to limit noise and visual distractions while working—that is, remove Spotify and work in deeper solitude with your noise-canceling headphones on.

Think Your Way to a Better Lupus Brain

Scientists once believed our brains were fixed and could not change. Now they know otherwise, as that big, beautiful brain of yours is a powerful learning machine. It's constantly reorganizing and rewiring itself based on what you're doing, thinking, and feeling, through a process called neuroplasticity. This is a good thing for an inflamed brain.

What Is Neuroplasticity?

Your brain can change many times over the course of your life in response to both internal and external events. The brain is highly malleable, allowing for the reprogramming of negative habits, the strengthening of beneficial neural connections, and overall improvement.

Because if circumstances can change, so can you. Your brain can change how it works and even how it looks in response to things like events, experiences, thoughts, and even emotions. Even if you feel like you are stuck in your ways, you can change. Neuroplasticity allows you to rewire that brain for less anxiety, more happiness, or more inner strength. The choice is yours here, and the possibilities feel practically endless.

Brain Habits

When you realize that certain thoughts or actions aren't serving you, you'll need to understand how to utilize the neuroplasticity processes of your brain.

Your brain naturally forms connections based on your habits and actions, and this process continues as you age. Whether it's worrying too much, seeing something as a positive over a negative, or even habitually scratching your head, these actions become ingrained in your brain over time. It is like how your dog will run in the same circle in the backyard until the grass wears down.

For example, if you had a painful blood draw from an inexperienced, masochistic lab tech, your mind would think, "Oh man, here comes the pain," at your next blood draw. After enough repetitions of this feeling, the brain's pathways become ready to trigger this reaction, even if that particular blood draw is painless. You see, the brain becomes a little too good at keeping you safe at times. It's so efficient that it can make you feel anxious when, in fact, you're actually going to be totally fine.

That's why breaking certain habits can be challenging. When you've been engaging in a specific action for a long time, your brain creates pathways that make it easier to continue that habit. It's easier to develop additional good habits if you already have a set of daily habits because your brain is wired to support them. On the other hand, breaking bad habits is harder once those pathways are established. However, it's important to remember that any action, thought, or habit, whether good or bad, can be created or broken with the right approach.

Retrain That Brain

One way to kickstart neuroplasticity is by learning new things or doing things that require the use of different skills. This opens the door to emotional and behavioral change while creating new, stronger neural connections.

Here are some ways to make that big brain stronger:

- At the start of the day, do the thing you've been dreading first.
- Learn something new, like growing your vocabulary and memory by reading, memorizing all the countries in the world, trying the cello, or talking to people who have different views than you.
- Break up the monotony of life by doing things in a different way. Drive a new route to work, change up your work routine, or order a new style of food to eat. Laotian food, anyone?
- Do everyday things with your nondominant hand, like brushing your teeth or eating with a fork or chopsticks (a way harder task).
- Travel more. It exposes your brain to new sights, smells, and sounds, opening up new neural pathways.

Oh yeah, it's best to try out these new techniques when your brain isn't already in mental fuckery mode.

Reflections

- NPSLE is a scary problem whose causes and treatment options remain largely unknown.
- Brain fog is a common mental symptom of lupus associated with stress, fatigue, diet, and more.
- Staying organized, making lists, and banning multitasking are ways to help with the fogginess.
- You can make improvements and rewire your brain by doing new things.

11

Lupus Mental Fuckery

Mental health problems don't define who you are. They are something you experience. You walk in the rain and you feel the rain, but you are not the rain.

—Matt Haig

During my first visit with my current rheumatologist, she said, "Have you noticed yourself feeling down this past year?" I was shocked to be asked this. For over a decade, I've received care for my autoimmune diseases, and no one ever asked about my mental health. It was as if this part of me wasn't as important as the physical side.

So, yeah, I was caught off guard when she asked this, and, due to my emotions being so raw, I whimpered out a yes. Because, man, it had been one shitty year. I spat on it and gave it the evil eye at the same time. I'd spent the majority of this year in physical and mental pain. One of my best girlfriends passed away from liver cancer. In her absence, I lost one of my biggest advocates and the strongest sources of positivity. My husband was running a business in another state and was traveling home every week, making it harder to connect with him. My youngest was in her second virtual school year, and this was wearing thin for both of us. During this year, I floated like a boat without a dock to anchor on.

This was the second year of COVID, and people were dying from the virus all over the world. And this made me feel like a big asshole, like I shouldn't even complain. Instead, I need to suck it up and stop feeling bad for myself. Sure, I was grateful for the health I had and for that of my family, but my current perspective kinda sucked. I just wanted to be healthier on all levels. Plus, I wanted all of that other crap in my life to, well, improve.

When my doctor asked me about depression and anxiety, it was like she opened the floodgates to address a piece of lupus that is typically stigmatized and hidden away. It's so shameful that your own doctors don't bring it up because it makes them uncomfortable and/or they lack the training and resources to guide you if you actually ask for their help.

Get ready for a mental health roller coaster in this chapter. We're diving deep into the wacky world of lupus and its effects on your sanity. Brace yourself for the notorious duo of depression and anxiety as they make their grand entrance. We'll also tackle the pesky shame that often tags along with mental health struggles, but fear not! You'll acquire an arsenal of steps you can take to find the support you need, no matter how big or small the craziness gets.

Mental Illness and Lupus

Did you know that individuals living with lupus are at a higher risk of experiencing depression and anxiety? It's a startling statistic that shows 25 percent of people with lupus experience depression, and 40 percent suffer from anxiety.[25] In the general population as a whole, only 3.8 percent of people have depression, and 19 percent have anxiety.

Living with lupus can be hard because of the physical symptoms, unpredictable flare-ups, and constant need to manage medications and appointments. Having to deal with these problems every day can be hard on a person's mental health. But why is it that people with lupus are more likely to have depression and anxiety?

First, the physical symptoms of lupus can make it more likely that a person will become depressed. Some medications used to treat lupus, like moderate to high levels of steroids, can upset the delicate balance of chemicals in the brain, which can cause mood changes and signs of depression. This risk can be made worse by stopping these kinds of drugs, which can make for a tough situation. It can also result from the extreme mental and emotional stress that comes with having this chronic disease.

SLE also has a big effect on one's quality of life that cannot be ignored. The illness can limit your mobility, cause constant pain, and drain your energy. This can make you feel frustrated, alone, and like you have lost something. Dealing with the unknowns and problems that come with lupus can be emotionally draining and make it easier to fall into depression.

Lupus can cause these mental health problems and symptoms directly, and it can also make them worse by making your quality of life crappier. This is kind of like being doomed, whether you do something or not.

You might have anxiety after receiving your SLE diagnosis and dealing with all the particulars that come along with lupus. Perfectly understandable. Or you might have anxiety as a result of lupus messing with the chemicals in your central nervous system.

In the end, it doesn't matter if lupus caused your anxiety or if it's a direct result of dealing with the disease. The fact remains that your anxiety is still there. Now, I've been going on about anxiety, but the same idea applies to depression. The end result is that you shouldn't feel guilty or like you've done something wrong to bring on this mental illness.

Severity and lupus

The intensity of one's mental health symptoms is not necessarily related to the severity or progression of SLE. Meaning that a woman with depression may not necessarily have a more severe lupus case than someone with a mild case of depression. This shows how important it is to treat both the physical and mental symptoms of SLE separately and to get the right care for both. Let's go a bit deeper to learn more about each of these mental illnesses.

Depression

Depression is the most common psychological problem among those with lupus, and it's way more than simply being sad. Depression is perpetual sadness without quite knowing the source of this feeling. It screams, "There's no point in doing anything because nothing will make a difference!" Depression is stolen confidence and awful thoughts. It's a total loss of who you are. It fucking sucks. It can make simple tasks, like making a meal, so challenging that no amount of positive thinking will ever make them go away.

Symptoms of depression

Having depression isn't always so obvious; know that it can show up as:

- canceling medical appointments, stopping medications, and not taking care of your health
- stopping activities you once enjoyed (exercising, socializing, sex, etc.)
- feeling fatigued or restless
- overeating or undereating
- sleeping too much or not enough
- difficulty concentrating and making decisions
- feeling guilty or worthless
- being irritable, easily frustrated, and increasingly nonfunctional

The World Health Organization finds that depression is the leading cause of poor health and disability and causes the greatest overall loss of functioning out of all disorders worldwide. I totally get this, as depression is so painful and debilitating on many levels. For some, depression can be more disabling than lupus.

Depression No-No

A lot of people throw around the word depression like it's just a normal feeling. "I am so depressed that Anthropologie didn't have those jeans in my size." Or "Ugh, I'm depressed that Auntie Anne's ran out of cinnamon sugar pretzels." Depression is a clinically diagnosable illness, not just a fleeting feeling or exclamation. If you are not clinically depressed, you might want to take this feeling out of your vocabulary. Instead, try the words hurt, disappointed, isolated, lonely, or sad. Please and thank you.

Anxiety

Anxiety is defined as "a state of full-body disequilibrium at a level of intensity that demands immediate attention and corrective action on your part," says author Faith Harper in Un fuck Your Brain. It feels like intense and excessive worry about everything. Anxiety is a combination of rational and irrational fear, a lack of hope, and a sense of impending doom that makes life so challenging. It is exhausting, unpredictable, and worsens at night.

How anxiety shows up is different for each person. For some, it feels like a heart attack, and you rush to the emergency department, certain you're dying, only to learn it's an anxiety attack. Another person may describe anxiety as living on a hamster wheel 24/7. No matter what, they can't get off, and it's impossible to ignore.

But hey, the good news is that you're not alone, as it's the most common mental health disorder in America. Thankfully, it's also the most treatable mental health illness—finally, a beacon of light in this darkness.

Symptoms of anxiety

Some signs of anxiety may include:

- excessive worrying
- being impatient, snappier than normal, or feeling misunderstood
- feeling like you are going crazy
- self-doubt
- compulsive and obsessive behaviors
- irrational fears and phobias
- trouble concentrating
- avoiding making future plans

Anxiety has a lot of physical symptoms that aren't always discussed. Light-headedness; headaches; muscle tension; trouble falling asleep; digestion problems (stomach issues, IBS, vomiting); pain in the chest, arms, legs, or back; numbness; and weakness are included in this list.

DON'T GIVE UP
HOPE
YOU
MATTER
YOU'RE NOT
ALONE

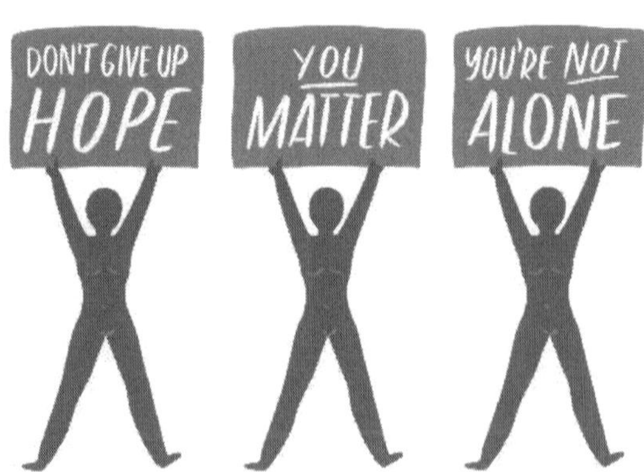

Getting the Help You Need

When does being nervous turn into anxiety? When does feeling sad turn into something serious like depression? Mental health can be hard to understand, but with professional help, a correct diagnosis, and treatment, you can get the support and relief you need. Getting the help you need takes on more urgency if you've noticed that your mental health is making your lupus worse.

Identifying mental health conditions

Recognizing the signs of a mental health problem can be the first step toward getting better. If you notice big changes in your thoughts, behaviors, or moods that last for more than two weeks and start to affect your work or relationships, it could be a sign of a mental health condition. Examples include missing important events, losing a job, or the breakup of a friendship.

It can be hard to tell the difference between normal emotional ups and downs and a possible mental health condition, especially if you feel intense emotions like sadness or worry all the time. It is important to remember that most mental health problems show up early in life, usually before the age of 25.

Seeking guidance

If you're worried about your mental health for any reason, reach out for help. Talk to your doctor, nurse, mental health professional, or a close friend or family member you trust who can help you get the help you need. Remember that problems with your mental health are medical issues that can affect your life just as much as problems with your physical health.

It is important to know that your worries do not have to be crippling before you can ask for help. No matter what is going on, your thoughts and feelings are real, and you deserve all the help you want and need.

Help ASAP

If you feel trapped by depression and/or anxiety and find your mind excessively worried or sad more often than not, get professional help. More serious symptoms need immediate attention.

It's time to get professional help right away if any of the following occur:

- any thoughts of self-harm or suicide
- persistent sleep issues
- feeling little to no enjoyment in the things you love
- feeling worthless
- isolating from others

Help finding help

Despite having access to the most mental health resources ever available, it remains quite a challenge to locate good mental health help (just like it is to find a good rheumatologist). Nationwide, there's a shortage of psychiatrists and counselors, plus limited inpatient psychiatric beds. Given this, you can expect a one-, two-, or three-month delay. Major bummer, I know! This explains why 6 percent of all emergency department visits are related to mental illness—people don't have access to treatments and seek immediate help when circumstances turn bleak.

Your primary care doctor (PCP) may be the first stop in this process. Even though they can technically diagnose mental disorders, PCPs typically do not have as much experience with mental health disorders as psychiatrists do. You may find that they'll listen to what is going on with you and, if necessary, suggest a prescription medication or refer you to a behavioral health practice.

A word of warning about large virtual mental health companies that offer quick diagnoses and what seems like easy access to depression and anxiety medications: Do your research before using such a company. Many large virtual mental health companies are getting more and more complaints about overprescribing medications after short evaluations by providers who don't have much experience with psychiatric diagnoses.

Treatment Options

The two most common types of mental illness treatment options include talk therapy and prescription medication. Sure, this won't fix everything you're going through, but it can help you get to a better place where you can manage your mental health.

Talk therapy

Counseling, or therapy, gives you a regular time and place to talk with a trained professional, usually a counselor or social worker, about your thoughts, feelings, and experiences. Anyone who wants it can get it, and you do not need a clinical diagnosis to do so. Counseling can help you heal from and cope with a specific illness, problem, or feeling more effectively.

Therapy can seem daunting and uncomfortable; after all, you're spilling your guts to some random person. This discomfort is often short lived as you deepen your relationship with your counselor. As you go through the therapy process, you should slowly start to feel better, gain more self-confidence, and be able to make better decisions about how to move forward.

There are many types of therapists out there to help, but not everyone will be the right fit for you. Don't abandon hope after trying out one therapist who was a wanker, because it's a very personal experience and may take a few tries to find the right person to work with. Keep going until you find someone you like talking to.

Even though most therapy is done one-on-one, you can also consider group counseling. Here, people living with similar mental illnesses or concerns get together, which is a great way to understand each other better and learn new ways to deal with problems. Anything from a faith-based group to a peer support group to a group under the direction of a professional can be considered group counseling. Use your group to talk about what is going on in your life and how you are feeling mentally and emotionally, and ask other members for advice.

Most Popular Therapy

Cognitive behavioral therapy (CBT) is the most common kind of therapy for anxiety and depression. It is a relatively short-term treatment that teaches you how your thoughts, feelings, and actions are connected. It also helps you learn skills to deal with any negative patterns that may be causing you trouble and teaches you how to act in healthier ways.

People with anxiety, depression, stress, or phobias have found this method helpful. It's also popular with people who want to stop unhealthy behaviors like smoking or eating too much.

Medication

Psychiatric drugs, in particular antidepressants, are often prescribed to help manage depression and anxiety in people with lupus. The goal of the medicines is to help you feel more mentally stable as you get your life back to a more normal routine. These drugs don't cure mental health problems, but they can ease the symptoms.

Like many other types of medications, antidepressants can be helpful in some situations but not in others. **Overall, antidepressants only help about 20 percent of people with their depression and anxiety.**[26] They are more helpful for people with chronic, moderate, or severe depression.[27] But they aren't as useful for mild depression.

Antidepressants can begin working in as little as seven days, but it could take several weeks to feel their full effect. In the meantime, be patient with your body as adjustments are made. Be aware that these medications can cause side effects that may mimic or intensify certain lupus symptoms, like sleep problems.

It's important to have regular appointments with your psychiatrist to review your symptoms, discuss any side effects, and adjust your dosage if needed. If one medication isn't working for you, don't fret. There are plenty of antidepressant options to try until the right one is found. Maintaining open and honest communication with your psychiatrist during this time will help you get the best medication.

My friend, do not lower your dose or stop taking the medication without alerting your doctor. Don't stop taking the antidepressants when you are feeling better, as they protect against your tendency to relapse. You wouldn't stop brushing your teeth because you didn't have a cavity after a year, right? This is the same as not stopping your medications just because your mind feels clearer. Also, it's best to slowly come off your drug dosage with your psychiatrist's permission and guidance. Stopping medications cold turkey can make withdrawal symptoms worse, and for some psychiatric medications, it can be dangerous.

Two-pronged approach

Antidepressants are not the be-all-end-all for removing your symptoms. Instead, psychiatrist Kiran Devaraj, MD, suggests viewing these medications as boosts of motivation toward positive mental health change. Think of it this way: if you need to climb over a tall wall, an antidepressant will serve as a leg up for you here. It won't push you over the edge—you've got to do this yourself—but it will make it easier to do it.

This is why therapy, when combined with pharmaceuticals, works well as a two-pronged approach for the treatment of depression, anxiety, and mental health illnesses, according to the American Psychological Association. Since therapy can also alter brain functioning for the better, it makes sense to combine antidepressants with it for maximum long-term benefits.

Mental Health Stigma

"It felt like all of my pain and my anxiety washed over me all at once, and it was one of the scariest times of my life. I sought support, and the doctors were able to give me a clear diagnosis. The moment that I received that emotion, I actually felt equal parts terrified and relieved. Terrified, obviously, because the veil was lifted, but relieved that I finally had the knowledge of why I suffered for so many years with depression and anxiety."

These were the words of Selena Gomez, who accepted an award for helping to remove the stigma associated with mental health. As a society, we often put more importance on physical health problems than mental health problems, and we forget how they affect people. It's absurd yet sadly accurate. The National Alliance on Mental Illness reports that 60 percent of adults do not receive necessary mental health care, largely due to the stigma surrounding it, which is downright ridiculous.

To be clear: people with mental illnesses are courageous warriors battling against their own minds and bodies to survive. They deserve empathy and respect, not shame and mockery. These stigmas are not only hurtful but also discourage people from getting help, leading to detrimental effects on their mental well-being, self-doubt, increased shame, and isolation.

Although we have made some progress in destigmatizing mental health thanks to influential figures like Selena Gomez, Naomi Osaka, and Kendrick Lamar, we still have a long way to go. It is important to raise awareness about mental health services, to reduce the shame that comes with getting help, and to make them easier to access and more affordable. But hey, at least we're taking baby steps in the right direction.

Reflections

- Ladies with lupus are at an increased risk of anxiety and depression.
- Get help if you are experiencing big changes in your thoughts, behaviors, or mood that last for more than two weeks.
- A combination of talk therapy and medication can be the best treatment for these conditions.
- People don't always get the help they need because of mental health stigma. This needs to change.

12

You. Emotional.

Our greatest asset in transforming the world and uplifting human dignity is healing ourselves so deeply that we become unwilling to harm others directly or indirectly.

—Unknown

It's been said that we learn more from losses than from failures. Well, I've discovered that this wisdom extends beyond achievements to include emotional journeys as well. Allow me to transport you back to 2019, when I lost a dearly loved one to a sudden death. It was the kind of loss that made me drop to my knees, sobbing, wondering why this happened and how I could go on without this person.

Thankfully, I was regularly practicing mindfulness at this time. The day after her death, I sat down to practice, closed my eyes, took one breath in and out, then started crying an ugly cry—the session was over. And over the next several days, I continued to show up and wail, although the crying fits decreased slowly. It felt as though my grief had a voice of its own, demanding to be acknowledged.

From this, I quickly understood why people turn to drugs, alcohol, or some other terrible vice in the face of powerful, painful emotions. The emotions that hurt so bad make you just want to get the hell away from them ASAP. Numbness could be a welcomed reprieve at times like this.

But this wouldn't allow me (or anyone else) to process the pain and grief. It would just keep me stuck where I was.

On this day, at this point in my life, I was grateful to be able to process what I was going through, to feel the sadness in my bones, and to give myself space to heal. I'm certain that it made the healing process easier and healthier, both at that moment and in the future.

Through the lens of loss, I have come to understand the incredible power of our emotional experiences. They shape us, teach us, and stretch the boundaries of our resilience. Even though the pain may be unbearable, it shows how much we can love and how strong we are when things do not go our way.

In this chapter, we explore the significance of emotions in our journey with lupus. Discover why all types of emotions, not just positive ones, hold importance. As we navigate the stages of grief, we draw parallels between a lupus diagnosis and the loss of a loved one. Let's untangle the complicated web of emotions and see how they can change us and help us grow emotionally despite the challenges of lupus.

Emotions Give Direction

Getting a lupus diagnosis is an emotional roller coaster. One minute you're thinking, "Okay, I've got this," and the next minute you're sobbing about how your pretty hair is in a pile on the floor.

Emotions are a big part of who we are and affect how we relate to other people and to ourselves. Look, everyone has feelings, even if they won't admit it. All feelings are normal and healthy, and everybody goes through hard ones. What matters is how you deal with them.

Think of your feelings as waves that rise and fall. They tend to get more intense over time, hit a peak, and then grow smaller. Surfing the emotional waves is easy enough when emotions are comfortable, but it's more challenging with hard emotions like uncertainty or jealousy.

Negative emotions are here to give feedback just as much as positive ones do. These hard feelings teach us important things about what we care about, who we trust, and how we want to live our lives. While fear (or guilt or jealousy) is totally normal, we shouldn't let it run our lives or keep us from doing things that are important. Stuffing feelings down or pushing them away only makes them stronger. Thankfully, feelings are temporary and pass, but they are more likely to stick around if they have a message to give us.

It's OK TO
Feel LIKe SHit
iM DOiNg It
RiGHt nOW

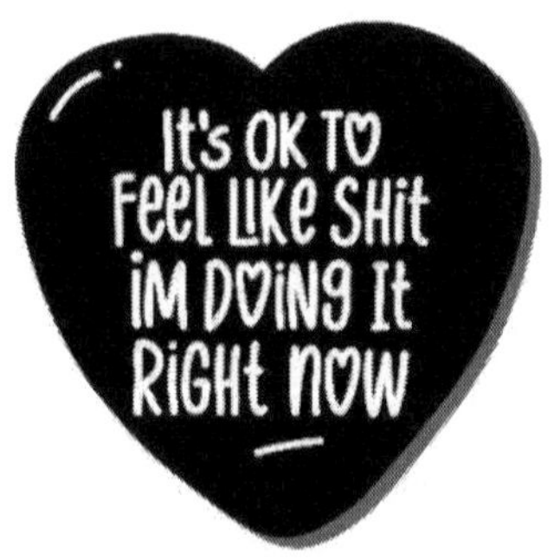

Alternatively, we can fight our feelings by avoiding or denying them. But this is not good for our mental health, and a lot of physical pain and suffering can come from this, both for yourself and your relationships.[28] What is going on at times like this is that we are escaping from our inner lives. Uncomfortable bodily sensations signal that emotions are brewing beneath the surface, setting us off, and we'd do anything to avoid facing them. Perhaps we can distract our minds by tackling sixteen things on the to-do list or by watching endless videos of dancing cats, but in the end, the emotions are still there, just waiting to be noticed.

According to Susan David, PhD, a psychologist and author of *Emotional Agility*, **feelings are guides, not directives**. That is, you do not have to act on your feelings. Instead, you should try to understand, accept, and express them.

Nothing can be changed until you're aware that you're doing it, so the first step is to observe what you're thinking about. What's going on inside that brings up this emotion? When a negative feeling comes up, David suggests giving it a name. Is it frustration, gloom, or annoyance? Why has this feeling shown up now? What's it trying to say?

Now that you know what is bothering you, try to come up with two more words that describe what you're feeling. This can bring up feelings that are buried and help you better understand what's going on internally.

Permit yourself to feel whatever it is you are feeling without judgment or the need to control it. Acknowledging and processing your emotions is essential, but it's equally important to not let these feelings control your decisions and actions. By taking a moment to consider how you actually want to respond before the words spill out of your mouth, you are less likely to say things you'll regret.

Toxic Positivity

We touched on gratitude a few chapters back. It's important, but constantly being grateful doesn't guarantee that you or your lupus will get better or that you'll feel happier, because **trying to force yourself to be happy all the time is total crap**. It just keeps you stuck in a cycle of denying your real emotions, which isn't good for your personal growth.

"We get it! We're supposed to constantly focus on the silver linings and believe that hard, bad, impossible things make us stronger. We call bullshit. We think you're plenty strong already. It's okay to feel exhausted by what's happening. You don't always have to be strong or even strive to be stronger."

—@Emandfriends [29]

Don't be afraid to feel frustration, disappointment, or any other emotion that comes up throughout the day. Don't judge yourself for feeling down sometimes. You don't have to fake feeling okay. Life can be tough and fucking unfair, and it's okay to rant and process it. In fact, it's healthier than bottling up your feelings and pretending like everything's just dandy. You'll never be able to completely get rid of negative thoughts and feelings, but that's not the point.

Instead of resisting or suppressing your emotions, take ownership of your feelings and develop healthy strategies to navigate and process them. See feelings as valuable tools for personal growth and self-improvement. By accepting and learning from your emotions, you can cultivate greater strength and resilience.

Grieve, Lady

Finding out you have an incurable chronic disease is like getting a terrible prize in a not-so-fun game show. It's a major loss that messes with your body, energy, looks, and the future you had imagined. Farewell, possibilities! Cue the dramatic music.

This loss brings along a gang of powerful emotions that demand to be heard. While there's no official rulebook on how to mourn the fact that you have lupus, the quest is uniquely yours. While others may accompany you, you will tread your own path at your own pace and confront your own challenges.

The emotional fallout from receiving such a devastating diagnosis is similar to the loss of a loved one. Grief is the process of letting go of deep sorrow. Healing takes place on a trajectory. It can't be controlled or planned out. Grief does not know how to tell time and cares less if it is a good idea to have a cry session or not.

According to Elisabeth Kubler-Ross' book, *Death and Dying*, there are five distinct phases in the grieving process. Understanding the emotions associated with each stage can assist you as you navigate from intense emotions toward a place of greater acceptance.

Know that this grief journey is not straightforward, and you may not necessarily progress through the stages of grief in order. Some may move from stage 1 to stage 4 and then circle back to stage 2. It's a forward and backward swing until you arrive at a point where you embrace your illness as well as its difficulties. This whole process may span a decade or a lifetime, and that's perfectly okay. It's also possible to fall back to an earlier stage during a flare-up, and again, it's completely normal. The key lies in cultivating self-acceptance, both for yourself and for your SLE.

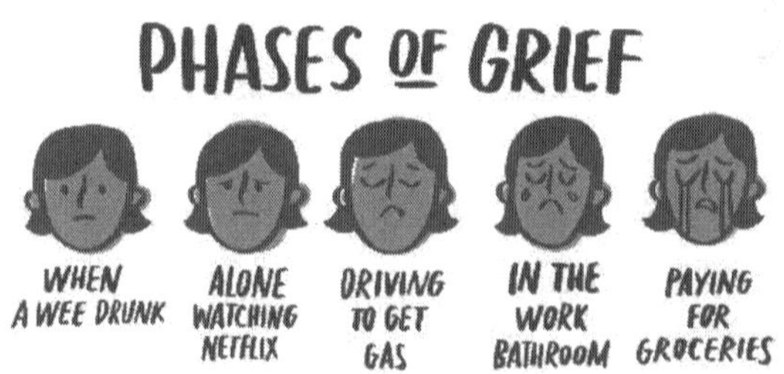

Stage 1: Shock

When you receive the official diagnosis, it's like a thunderbolt striking your world, leaving you in a state of shock. Denial becomes your best friend as your mind plays out worst-case scenarios. It's official: the shit has hit the fan.

In the midst of this chaos, you find yourself swimming in a sea of overwhelming emotions. The weight of what lies ahead and the long-term implications of your health situation may feel like a massive boulder on your chest. Your mind, in a desperate attempt to shield itself, puts up the Closed for Renovations sign, shutting down as a protective measure.

In this whirlwind of emotions, it's important to acknowledge that your ability to absorb information might resemble a leaky bucket. You might only catch a tiny portion of what you're being told during the diagnosis. Tapping into deeper levels of patience with yourself here is helpful, as is bringing along a family member who can take notes on what's being said.

Stage 2: Anger

During this stage, you transform into an anger-fueled force to be reckoned with, and boy, do you have every right to be pissed. Your life has taken an unexpected detour, and you find yourself drowning in a sea of thoughts like, "Why the hell did this happen to me?" or "Seriously, I can't even rent a damn car, yet I have a chronic disease?" The frustration runs deep as you grapple with the reality of having to alter your entire way of living. You even catch yourself blaming that extra Costco hot dog or one too many gel manicures as the trigger for your lupus, as if fate had it out for you.

Simultaneously, your anger extends beyond yourself, reaching outward toward your significant others and loved ones. You can't help but feel pissy about the insensitive things they say or do. Deep down, there's a part of you that secretly resents them for not bearing the burden of lupus in your place. It's easier and somewhat safer to direct your anger at them because they're your loved ones, and they'll stick around even when you unleash snarky comments like, "Oh, it must be SO wonderful to be all shiny and healthy!"

Your anger reaches celestial heights as you find yourself fuming at Mohammed, Jesus, Jehovah, Buddha, or even the whole damn universe for bestowing SLE upon you. After all, you've strived to be a decent human being throughout your lifetime, spreading kindness like confetti and recycling like a champion. Doesn't all that good karma count for something?

But here's the secret, my fiery friend. Your anger serves a purpose in your healing journey. When you shift from feeling powerless and asking,

"Why me?" to defiantly declaring, "Fuck you, lupus! I deserve better," you reclaim your power. It's a moment of pure magic when you seize control of your SLE instead of allowing it to dictate your life.

Stage 3: Bargaining

In this phase of grief, bargaining becomes your go to strategy as you attempt to wrestle control away from lupus. You find yourself making all sorts of deals and pacts, like saying, "I'll dedicate my entire life to saving the endangered mole rat of Peru if my doctor's diagnosis turns out to be wrong."

You see, bargaining happens all the time. It's the "if, then" scenarios we run through to get what we want, like in middle school when you prayed for your boobs to finally grow.

You meticulously consider every possible scenario, desperately seeking a way to regain your health. But no matter how many deals you make or how carefully you weigh the outcomes, the end result remains unchanged. You've got lupus. You can't get rid of it. It's attached to you forever, and that's a long-ass time.

Stage 4: Sadness

During this fourth phase, you may find yourself overwhelmed by feelings of sadness, helplessness, and hopelessness. It's as if a heavy weight settles in your mind and trickles down to every cell in your body. Headaches and stomachaches are common during this time. It's common to cry a lot here, so let those tears come. It's understandable to feel deep sadness when moving forward, and making decisions feels incredibly challenging.

It's helpful to find a path or outlet to lighten the load at this time, whether from a counselor or a trusted friend. Remember, you don't have to face these emotions alone, and there are resources available to help you navigate this diagnosis and regain your inner strength.

Stage 5: Acceptance

Welcome to the acceptance stage of having lupus, where the clouds begin to part and you catch glimpses of light shining through. It's not a full rainbow yet, but you can see the potential ahead. This stage is both the healthiest and the most challenging in the grief process.

To thrive, you must accept what you can't control and acknowledge what you have. **Lupus is a part of you, but it doesn't define you.** It's just a piece, like your freckles or the mole on your left shoulder. You can have lupus and still be so much more.

You have the choice to change your mindset from seeing lupus as an all-consuming bad thing to seeing it as something you have that doesn't have you. Don't waste your life wishing it was easier—this will only delay your progress. Work on becoming better, stronger, and smarter. The most badass version you can cultivate. Be open to the changes that occur in your body and mind. While it's not easy, forcing yourself to remain the same doesn't benefit you like acceptance does. Give yourself grace and compassion as you enter this roller coaster of a life with lupus.

The less you fight your diagnosis, the better your life will be. See yourself in a transitional phase, gathering tools, knowledge, and wisdom for the next chapter. And that takes a moment (or two or three) to develop. Trust the timing of your life, and trust your inflamed, resilient body to navigate through this.

Reflections

- All emotions are important, not just the positive ones.
- Work on understanding, accepting, and expressing your emotions.
- Being diagnosed with lupus is a grieving process that happens in stages.
- Understanding what happens at each stage can help you move from shock to acceptance.

13

Vaginas, Uteri, and Preggers, Oh My!

If I say I'm beautiful . . . if I say I'm strong, you will not determine my story—I will.

—Amy Schumer

When it comes to my first pregnancy, I like to consider myself lucky. Little did I know that while I was busy growing a tiny human inside me, lupus was secretly setting up camp in my cells, like uninvited guests who overstay their welcome. Pregnancy turned out to be the catalyst for my lupus journey, and boy, did it make its grand entrance in style.

I must admit, looking back, it's quite comical how clueless I was about what was brewing in my body. The word lupus never even made it onto my pregnancy radar. Despite the unexpected surprise, I managed to survive the wild ride and deliver a feisty little daughter who will undoubtedly leave her mark on this world.

So yes, I like to think of myself as lucky, in a twisted sort of way. I am lucky to have survived the pregnancy and even luckier to now be a mom with lupus who gets to support a daughter who also has lupus. It's like a twisted two-for-one deal, where the price of bringing a new life into the world included a chronic illness subscription for both parties. Talk about getting more than you bargained for.

But hey, I'm learning to embrace the unexpected. Life has a funny way of throwing curveballs at us, and I've become quite good at dodging them with style and grace (or at least attempting to). So here I am, rocking the mom lupus daughter combo like a badass with a sidekick disease that's equal parts shitty and infuriating.

By now, it should come as no surprise that lupus can even impact your gynecological, reproductive, and sexual health. What part of the body doesn't SLE damage, you ask? I'm still looking and will get back to you on this. In the meantime, this chapter will share some challenges that you may face here. It's important to know how lupus may show up in your vagina, uterus, and all the other reproductive areas so you can be armed with knowledge, and then you can add in some prevention to be prepared when issues do arise.

Gynecological Issues

Your uterus, ovaries, fallopian tubes, endometrium, vagina, vulva, and cervix are all part of your gynecological system. Since most women are diagnosed between the ages of 15 and 45, your period, sex, and choosing the right birth control have different effects on you than they do on healthy women. Here are the most common ways that lupus affects your gynecologic system.

Painful periods

Does your period feel like you got hit by a truck since you were diagnosed? If so, welcome to the club. Lupus isn't just a party pooper; it can also disrupt your menstrual cycle and turn your uterus into a war zone. And don't even get me started on the ovulation issues caused by chronic inflammation and stress—it's like your ovaries are going through a midlife crisis. Cramps can come on stronger, and at times, it feels like your period won't stop.

Be conscious that being in a flare and on your period at the same time can make you feel exponentially worse. Now, is it lupus's fault? Or is it your period's problem? It's hard to tell exactly, but they do affect one another.

Your period can be mistaken for a lupus flare because there is so much gray area between where one symptom of lupus begins and where it ends. For example, your headaches may be a result of stress and inflammation, but they could also be PMS. Or from the flare that your body is entering. Hell, maybe it's all of these things.

Your period can also increase flare symptoms. When you add this to an already pissed off lupus body, you better watch out. Recently, it felt like one of my ovaries burst in pain when I was in a very bad flare and on my period. It was one of the most painful periods to date, and I even considered going to the ER.

Take note: If you are using steroids to manage your inflammation, your risk for menstrual abnormalities, like irregular periods, increases. This is just temporary, and your cycle should return to normal when the medications are stopped.

Anemia

Anemia is a common sidekick of lupus. This is where your iron levels are low, and it can make you feel tired, thirsty, and moody—basically, like a hangry toddler. And if you're on your period, it's like a scene from Carrie, but with more pain and less telekinesis.

Yeast infections

Women with lupus are more prone to yeast infections—oh joy! Blame this on suppressed immunity. Yeast thrives in a moist, warm environment. When bacteria get in, the vaginal microbiome (did you even know there was such a thing?) isn't strong enough to kill it off. Hello, itching, burning, and redness. To combat it, it helps us to stay out of those tight leggings and nylon undies. Let your v-jay breathe with cotton panties and wear loose pants—that's right, rock the mom jeans.

UTIs

Be aware that you are at risk of being misdiagnosed with a urinary tract infection (UTI) when what you really could be developing is a kidney disease, a known symptom of SLE. When a urine sample is taken from a woman with SLE suspected of having a UTI, white and red blood cells appear in the culture. To a doctor who doesn't know her patient's history or understand lupus, it might appear as if it's a UTI. Do not accept a UTI diagnosis without a culture being run to check for bacterial growth.

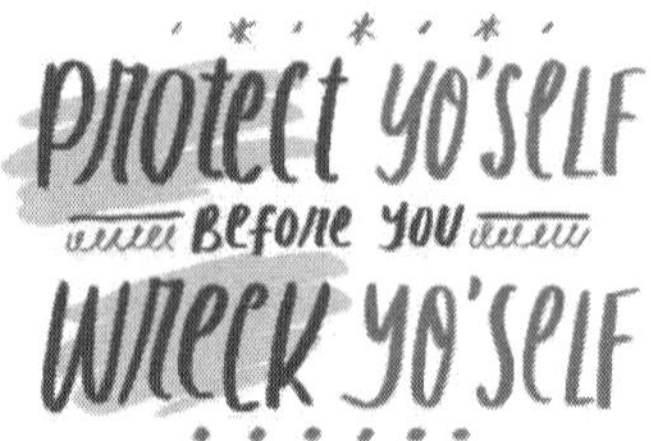

STIs

You need to be aware of the increased risk of three particular sexually transmitted infections (STIs). These include herpes and syphilis. If you've had herpes in the past, the use of immunosuppressant drugs can reactivate the virus after it's been dormant in your body. This results in a new herpes outbreak.

Roughly 20 percent of women with SLE test positive for syphilis. This occurs because the antibodies generated are very similar to those generated by a female fighting syphilis, leading to a false positive result. Even though you may have similar antibodies, this does not indicate that you have syphilis. It can be challenging for a physician to distinguish between syphilis and lupus, at least in the beginning phases of your disease.

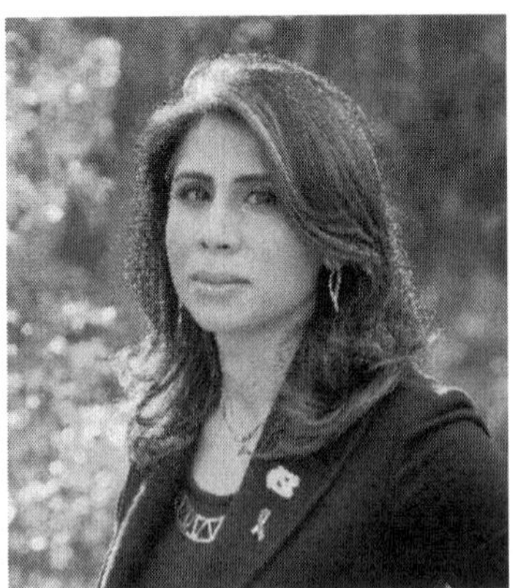

Interview with a Rheumatologist

Dr. Saira Z. Sheikh is a nationally renowned physician, researcher, and educator. She is trained and triple board certified in Internal

Medicine, Rheumatology, and Allergy/Immunology. Dr. Sheikh is the director of the clinical trials program at the UNC Thurston Arthritis Research Center, as well as the UNC Rheumatology Lupus Clinic. She serves on the American College of Rheumatology's board of directors, the Medical and Scientific Advisory Council of the Lupus Foundation of America, and is the current vice-chair of the Lupus Clinical Investigators Network. Moreover, she is my rheumatologist. Hurrah!

Dr. Sheikh would offer the following words of wisdom to a female patient who has recently been diagnosed with lupus.

1. **Allow yourself to feel** what you feel. It can feel frightening and overwhelming. Lupus can feel incredibly unfair and disruptive to your life, plans, and dreams. Know that it's okay to feel upset and frustrated, all of which are emotions that come with learning to cope with a chronic illness. Remember that it's important to allow yourself to recognize, acknowledge, and validate those feelings before rushing to move past them.
2. **Listen to your body**. If you don't feel right or think that something isn't working well for you, communicate with your doctor. It's important to ask questions and have a clear understanding of what to expect from the disease as well as the medications you are prescribed. This is a partnership, and you can be most successful in achieving your health goals when you work closely with your doctor.
3. **Feel empowered to advocate** for yourself—know that at any given time, YOU are the expert on your lived experience.

When the discussion turned to what's on the horizon for lupus, Dr. Sheikh responded, "The hope is that someday soon, we will have even safer and more effective therapies that are tailored to the specific needs of each individual, and this will allow our patients with lupus to live healthier and longer lives—for patients not just to survive but truly to thrive with lupus!"

Birth Control

The risks you face from getting pregnant at the wrong time are very significant for your lupus and your overall health. Find an OB/GYN who has knowledge of lupus and knows how it can impact your situation. It's critical to talk to your gynecologist about the right contraceptives, the potential risks, and the benefits. It is absolutely essential that you are vigilant about using a birth control method and take it exactly as prescribed.

In general, 10–20 percent of all women, not just those with SLE, may not be able to use combined hormonal contraceptives because of their specific medical condition, the severity of their disease activity, or certain conditions. Certain lupus medications reduce the effectiveness of your birth control. Other lupus drugs have side effects that can cause serious birth defects, demonstrating that it's imperative that you practice safe sex each and every time.

Preggers

Even for the healthiest of women, pregnancy is no easy task. Thankfully, the majority of women with lupus can have happy, healthy pregnancies where both mom and baby thrive.

Knowing that 50 percent of all pregnancies are unintended (I have one of those oops babies myself), it's essential that you plan out your pregnancy in advance and don't leave it to chance. This means you shouldn't stop taking any birth control until you are 100 percent ready to conceive.

You want to enter pregnancy as the healthiest version of yourself. Ideally, your SLE will be stable, and flares will be low to nonexistent. Being strong mentally and physically will put you in the best position for your unborn baby and yourself.

Most women with SLE do not have any extra problems when they try to get pregnant. If you are missing periods or aren't having periods at all due to a high disease activity state, this is an important consideration because you need a period to get pregnant. Also, if you have kidney disease, this can make it harder (and riskier) to conceive.

To have the safest pregnancy possible, start with open and honest conversations with your obstetrician and rheumatologist to assess your risks, review medications, and get guidance on the best way to move forward before getting pregnant. You can assume some compromises will need to be made during pregnancy, and you will be considered high-risk. Don't sweat it, though. This just means they will take extra special care of you.

By far, the majority of babies born to women with lupus are born healthy and will not have lupus. Statistics show that between 1 and 3 percent of babies born to mothers with SLE will have lupus.[30]

With careful planning, your chances of having a happy, healthy pregnancy and a happy, healthy baby are very high. Give it careful consideration, and don't rush into the situation without discussing it with your OB/GYN and rheumatologist.

Reflections

- Gee, thanks, lupus, for worming your way into a woman's most private parts.
- SLE can bring a bunch of things you don't want, like UTIs and yeast infections.
- Please, please stay on birth control until you're 100 percent ready to have a baby.
- Most women with lupus can have healthy, happy pregnancies where both mother and child do well.

14

Get Those Orgasms and Sexy Time Back

Life is like sex. It's not always good, but it's always worth trying.

—Pamela Anderson

Lupus has done a number on your sex life. Gotcha! I can totally relate. This is where my husband sighs heavily and says I reveal too much. Having both lupus and Sjogren's, my lady parts have suffered along with me. The dryness made sex painful, fatigue rocked my world, and my throbbing joints consumed my thoughts. Sex was the last thing on my mind.

But I understood that it's an important part of my life and my husband's, plus it's an extension of our relationship, a way to connect with him on a deeper level, and it just feels good. That's why I was concerned and perplexed as to why sex got harder. My rheumatologist never mentioned the possibility that sex would shift after my autoimmune diagnosis. In fact, it was only after a doctor's Google search that I discovered what was going on.

Thankfully, with some knowledge and relatively simple actions, I was able to take charge of my situation and manage the impact lupus has on my sex life. While I understand that it's an ongoing, evolving process, I'm grateful that this is one area of lupus that I can control for now. My husband is happy too—he just won't come out and say it, you know, because it's way too revealing.

Prepare for some sexy talk in this chapter. You'll learn about how lupus challenges your sexual health and ways you can combat it. You'll learn why an orgasm a day keeps your rheumatologist away, how exactly to do this, and how to find solutions to your sex challenges that work.

Sex Challenges

Sex is important, and it should feel good. It's a great way to let off some steam. It also makes you more relaxed, and it does your body good. Endorphins, known as nature's pain reliever, are released during sex. Studies show that **your immune system grows stronger with sex**. "All right, all right, all right," says Matthew McConaughey. When a couple has a good sexual life, they feel closer to each other and are less likely to fight or blame each other.

Having a healthy, happy, intimate sex life is essential for women with lupus. Hell, I'm pretty sure it's important for all human beings who are sexually active. So what's the problem? It's that damn lupus again. With a chronic disease, sexual dysfunction is more common than you think. There is no denying that the physical, emotional, and mental effects of SLE can impact your relationships, intimacy, and sexuality.

Reasons for Sex Pain

Chronic pain, major joint stiffness, low self-esteem, exhaustion, and a host of other factors can make sex a miserable experience for women living with SLE.

A few other ways lupus can get in the way of good sex:

- vaginal ulcers*
- mouth ulcers
- limited range of motion in hips, knees, and other joints
- yeast infections and/or UTIs
- emotional roadblocks

*Compared to oral ulcers, vaginal sores and ulcers are rather uncommon, thankfully.

Your desire for sex is tied to your disease activity as well, meaning **the more severe your lupus is, the more sexual problems are likely to occur**. All of these components affect how good or bad you feel about being intimate with your partner and getting your sexy on.

Dry V-Jay

Ever tried to insert a tampon into a perfectly dry vagina? It hurts just as much, if not more, to have sex when your vagina is dry. It's like shoving your arm into one of those pool arm floaties—owie! A lupus symptom or the dryness brought on by the medications used to treat the condition may hurt your poor lupus vagina.

Take heart, though. There are options out there to make this more bearable. It just takes a little bit of lubricant to make a big difference. Stick to a natural, non-water-based lube, like the one my friend gave me that was CBD-infused. (Yeah, that is one good friend right there!) Use a bunch of it each time. Stay away from petroleum jelly because it can encourage bacterial and yeast growth. If a lubricant isn't working, consider a visit to your gynecologist for an open discussion about creams or other medications that can help a girl out.

Emotional roadblocks

To be real, even on a good day, a woman's sense of self-worth can rise and fall for a variety of reasons. All of this has an impact on how you feel and think about yourself, especially when it's time to get naked.

Lupus can bring about significant bodily changes, like losing or gaining weight, due to ongoing inflammation and swelling. And a lot of these changes suck, and you seriously want them to fuck off, but instead, they stick around, like the hair loss and the bright red rash on your face. When pain and weariness set in, your beauty routine may start to take on less significance.

Lupus, in turn, makes it harder to understand your body and messes with your mind and how you view yourself. It's the negative self-talk that makes you doubt yourself, how you look, and your abilities. When you aren't feeling particularly confident and self-assured, you probably won't feel like being intimate.

Embarrassing for All

Sexual intimacy and intercourse are the two topics most often overlooked and avoided in healthcare discussions. Most doctors simply do not have the time (or, let's be real, the insurance codes) to ask these questions. Plus, a lot of additional training is needed on sexuality and intimacy, as many healthcare providers don't know how to approach these topics and concerns.

Age, spiritual beliefs, race, and fear are some factors that may keep you from openly discussing this topic with your provider. But rest assured, your sex challenges are perfectly legitimate things to talk about with your rheumatologist, gynecologist, PCP, and therapist—even if it remains embarrassing to do so.

Meds affecting sex

Common lupus medicines can impact your gynecological health, and they leave you vulnerable to infections that cause pain and discomfort down there. Yeast infections are one type of infection that can make sex unappealing, especially when you have to use vaginal suppositories. However, infections are not the only health threat. The disruption of hormones by medication can cause a wide range of side effects, including changes in mood, energy, and focus

But wait, there's more! Steroids are the go-to medication to bring people out of a flare-up, but they can also mess with your mind, make it harder to sleep, and even make you feel angry or anxious. Needless to say, sex isn't a top priority at this time. On top of that, some medications, like antidepressants and blood pressure drugs, can lower your libido, making it even more challenging to get in the mood. While these drugs can be incredibly helpful in managing lupus symptoms, it's essential to be aware of their potential side effects on your sexual and gynecological health.

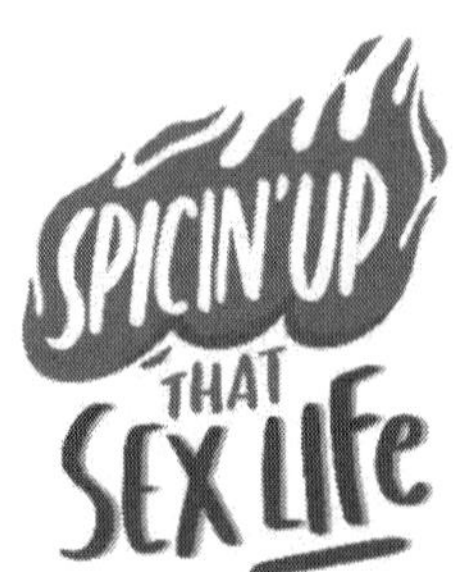

Sexy Solutions That Work

Whether it's through the symptoms you experience from SLE, the side effects of the medications you are on, or the lost drive from the whole shitshow, lupus can impact your sex life. You're going to have to put in a little more effort when it comes to sex and your relationship with your partner, just like you have to with everything else in your life now that you have lupus.

Think of it this way. The alternative is to accept that you are stuck watching Bridgerton on repeat to kick your sexual libido into high gear. Or maybe you're considering a vow of abstinence because you've convinced yourself that sex really isn't that important. Hell no! Don't give up hope—there's a way to boost your intimacy so that sex is more enjoyable. There are options available to you, but they will involve a bit of creativity, a dash of patience, and the ability to clearly communicate your needs to your partner.

Review Your Symptoms

First things first, look at what is stopping you from having sex. This is where joint pain, mouth ulcers, tiredness, medications, and other symptoms make it more challenging to enjoy sex or have it as often as you'd want to. The key here is to develop a deeper awareness of your body and pay attention to the details and signs before things spiral out of control.

Figure out the specific problem(s) you are having when it comes to sex. Make a list of what's stopping or hurting you, and be completely honest with yourself. Is it that your hip throbs so much that sex has become unbearable? Are you worried about what your partner thinks of you now that you have lupus? Is it the extra weight you've put on since starting that new round of steroids that's stopping you from initiating sex?

Check your med(s)

Read up on your medication's side effects. Look up unfamiliar words and phrases; for example, "atrophic vaginitis" is the medical term for vaginal dryness.

Cross-reference this against your sex-stopper symptoms from above. Does your medication explain the extra tiredness? Is your new anti-anxiety drug list responsible for the low libido? Knowing how your lupus medicines work can help you figure out what's going on in your body.

Take some action

Do something with the information you've gathered. Talk to your rheumatologist, OB/GYN, or prescriber if you have a drug side effect that's treating you poorly. Perhaps an alternate drug is available or additional solutions can be provided to lessen your barriers.

Do you experience pain during sex that a drug's side effects cannot account for? If so, bring this up with your gynecologist. Don't forget that your doctors are sexual beings who also happen to be trained doctors. They care about your overall health and will work with you to make it better. You'll have to push through embarrassing feelings and be honest about what you're going through.

Do you have limited movement in your shoulder that is stopping you from getting it on? Go see a physical therapist (PT) and work on the issue. Some people can self-refer to a PT, but check with your insurance company first. Yes, your physical therapist has had sex before, so there's no need to be awkward about bringing up this issue.

If it's not a medication issue but rather an emotional and mental health concern, let's get ya some outside help. There are so many great resources to consider, from a self-help book to a webinar to therapy. There are even sex education therapists ready to guide you toward a more satisfying sexual relationship. You've got to take the first step, though, to get help.

The Big "O"

An orgasm a day keeps the rheumatologist away. Wait, did I lose you? Did you roll your eyes? Hold on. There's some good stuff here. Trust me: read on.

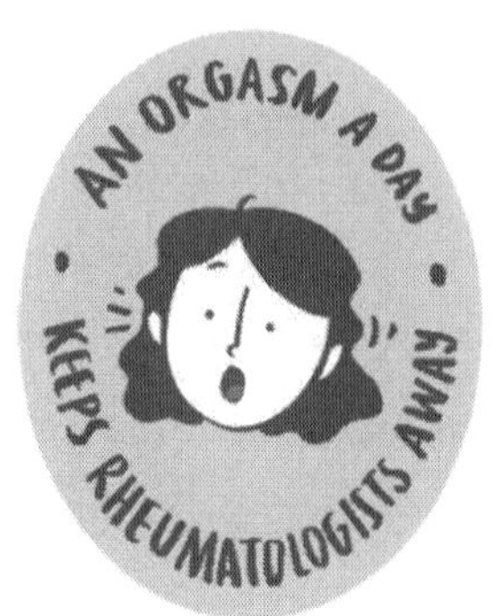

When you have an orgasm, pleasure hormones spew through your body. Dopamine and oxytocin, to be exact. These hormones temporarily make you feel great, relaxed, and happy while your heart thumps, you get flushed and sweaty, and your blood pressure goes up. **You see, an orgasm is a full body workout.**

It's good for the entire body. In the Rutgers Orgasm Lab, Barry Komisaruk, PhD, discovered that orgasms are nature's painkillers, with up to a 50 percent decrease in pain being experienced. It's not surprising because an orgasm is a healthy release of muscle tension. But there are even more perks, including:

- reduced stress and tension
- improved sleep
- boosted body image
- decreased menstrual pain
- improved circulatory, neural, and muscular systems

As a result of this burst of relaxation and clarity, you feel better inside and out.

Fine, fine, you say to the daily orgasm idea, and now you're wondering how the hell to do just this. You've got two choices: sex or masturbation. Also, only 18 percent of women have the ability to climax with sexual penetration.[31] And masturbation is the easiest one because: (1) you don't need a partner; (2) you can't get pregnant; and (3) there's no threat of a sexually transmitted infection. Woot, woot—bring on the orgasm.

Step 1: Get in the Mood

Find the best time to masturbate when you don't have obligations and no one will interrupt you. Choose a location that is equally cozy and private. Maybe that's at night or when your home is empty. Get in the mood by reading a naughty book, lighting some candles, or turning on some sexy music.

Step 2: Get Out of Your Head and into Your Crotch

Be intentional about why you're taking time to pleasure yourself. Think of the good stuff that comes along with an orgasm, like how you'll feel more relaxed and sleep better. Focus on the pleasure about to be experienced. Don't feel pressured to have an orgasm every time. Simply enjoy.

Step 3: Get Down to Business

Bow chicka wow wow-grab your non-water-based lube and get to work with either your fingers or a sex toy (whether that be a vibrator, dildo, or vibrating wand). Don't be shy: you're in good company. Half of all US females use a vibrator for orgasm because they are consistently reliable and much easier to get off with. This means bring on the toys, my friend.

Step 4: Savor the Afterglow

After that orgasm, take a few minutes to relax and bask in the afterglow. Think of this as the savasana, or resting phase, done at the end of a yoga session. Don't jump up and start doing something. Relish as those good vibes (and hormones) surge through you.

Keeping relationships sexually healthy

Just so you know, this sex stuff isn't all about you if you're in a relationship, because your SLE affects your partner too. Basically, there are many ways lupus can place extra pressure on an existing relationship and have trickle-down effects in the bedroom. Your partner may be clueless about what actions to take to help you feel better. Your partner might be scared of hurting you during sex, so tread lightly in the boudoir (a fancy French word for the bedroom). Plus, lupus is unpredictable, so your partner won't know how you're feeling on any given day.

Assuming you still want to have sex, here are some ways to make it more fun and less painful:

- Take pain medicine an hour before having sex.
- Use pillows placed in the right spot to help ease painful joints during sex.
- Try out different sex positions to find ones that hurt less.
- Take a short nap before sex to feel rested and energized.
- Try sex in the morning or afternoon if you are too tired at night.
- Watch a sexy show or read a sexy book beforehand. (*Fifty Shades of Gray*, anyone?)
- Try a change of scenery (a different room or hotel room).

Understandably, turning down your partner for sex can bring up some hurt feelings. Assumptions may arise from your partner about these declines, like, "Hmm, she doesn't find me sexy AF anymore." Your partner may think you don't care about his or her needs. What's a woman to do here? Here are two suggestions for you: (1) learn to express your sexual needs more clearly, and (2) take action to boost your intimacy.

Communicate, um, better

Good communication is the key to breaking down walls, getting closer, and improving your relationship. When you let your partner know what you're feeling, he or she will be better able to understand your emotional state and how to best help you.

Be open and fill your partner in on what's really going on with you. As my husband likes to remind me, he's not a mind reader. Unless I tell him exactly what I need, he will not be able to oblige. Talk about fantasies and desires. Lay it all on the table. You'll get the most bang for your buck when you discuss your needs outside of the bedroom, when tension is low and the risk of a fight is diffused.

Give direction

Having a solid intimacy plan and reasonable goals will help you turn your wants into doable actions. To defuse any potential fights, make statements that pertain to you alone and not about what your partner is or isn't doing. These "I" statements help you take responsibility for your feelings. Instead of "You suck at getting me off," which turns a bad situation worse quickly, opt for "I like it when you kiss my neck." Other examples of "I" statements include:

- I feel good when you do this…
- Let's try…
- It hurts me when…
- I like it when…
- My favorite place to be touched is this…

Deal with issues immediately

If there's an issue, don't avoid it and just hope that it'll all go away. This just builds up resentment and results in hurt feelings. Plus, it could put a crack in the relationship. Instead, it's helpful to bring up a concern as soon as you can. If there's pain during sex, talk about it and come up with a solution or two. Not feeling sexy tonight? Take a pause and let your partner know why you feel this way, so blame isn't internalized.

Alternatives to sex

Let your partner know that saying no to sex doesn't have to mean that you don't feel well enough for any hanky panky. Are you wanting no intercourse but still wishing to get some affection and connection from your partner?

- Snuggle, kiss, and make out like you're in high school.
- Give each other massages, but let your partner massage you first.
- Bring on sex toys without the promise of sex and just enjoy.
- Hold hands, sit close, hug, and touch each other.

Having a break from sex is okay, too. Take it off the table entirely. You'll have to relay the message to your partner that saying no to sex doesn't mean you think he/she is undesirable, and that he/she is still a sexy hunk of cheese (or whatever food you totally love) and 100 percent wanted by you. It's just a temporary thing until you feel better.

Reflections

- Lupus can cause many different kinds of sexual problems, and it is important to look into all of them.
- Consider an orgasm if you're looking for a quick way to reduce pain.
- You can keep your relationship sexually healthy with open, honest conversation.
- No to sex doesn't mean all forms of intimacy are off the table.

15

Stop Stressin' So Much, Friend

These mountains that you are carrying,
you were only supposed to climb.
—Najwa Zebian

I lost 10 percent of my body weight without trying. Now you're like, "Girl, don't hold out on me. Tell me what you did to make this happen." Happy to share. It's simple: I experienced a shitload of stress in a short period of time. Pounds magically dropped off. If you eat when stressed, this plan may backfire on you. I, on the other hand, forget to eat when overwhelmed because my mind is busy scheming, planning, and whirling with possibilities.

At this time, I was managing a huge, multimillion-dollar project involving the coordination of forty-plus independent contractors. My responsibilities involved a crapload of tasks that overloaded an already compromised brain.

When I first noticed my weight loss, I thought, "Oh, this is a nice surprise," and put my head back down to work. A few weeks passed, and the pounds kept dropping. Friends started asking me why I'd gotten thinner—this was their way of saying, "Eat something, please!" At the same time, errors were being made at work. I paid one person incorrectly and gave another person wrong information. In my head, it was getting harder and harder to keep all the logistics organized.

Since this crap was getting more serious, I looked into it. My rheumatologist said my labs were fine, so lupus, for once, wasn't to blame. There was nothing else to explain what was going on except my work stress. The ironic part was that I was running stress reduction training for businesses and teams, and I knew that not all stress is bad stress, yet I'd let this stress become bad. With this in mind, I got down to the work of taking care of myself again, mentally, physically, and spiritually. Because clearly, I needed help.

What if I told you that stress can actually be good for you and your lupus? Yeah, I know, mind blown, right? Small mental changes can make a big difference in dealing with the pressures of stress. The secret isn't to avoid all stress (as if you could), because the right kind can be motivating and good for your health. Understanding the difference is key. This chapter digs deep into the idea of stress and how it affects you.

Stress Explained

Stress is the way the body responds to changes. Whether it's physical or mental, if something is pressing, pulling, compressing, or twisting your body, it's causing stress. Imagine sitting in a sauna—the heat is stress. Or having someone knock on your door at 2 a.m.—yeah, that's definitely stressful.

Now, there's this other definition of stress that I love from Kelly McGonigal's book, *The Upside of Stress*. She defines stress as "what arises when something you care about is at stake." I can totally get behind this idea. This view puts stress into a new perspective and can make you wonder if you're stressing about things that you really care about. Sometimes the answer is yes, and connecting with the importance of this cause can energize you. Other times, it's a big fat no, and you can let that shit go.

Everyone Be Stressin'

Seriously, stress is like the doom and gloom of our society, and everyone is stressed to the max. **No one in this big, beautiful world is immune to the pressure of stress.** No matter how old you are, how much money you have, or how famous you are, stress won't go away.

Women know stress. Extreme stress affects women twice as often as men. We take it personally (thinking we did something wrong) and are more likely to do something to alleviate it, which is great. On the flipside, women are more likely to have mental health problems like depression or anxiety that get worse when stressed.

Great expectations

Stress can happen when your expectations are different from what happens in real life. Having such fixed ideas about how one's life should go makes a situation even more stressful. After being married for a few months, I asked my mom why she hadn't told me that marriage was so hard. She laughed and asked, "What made you think it was easy?" For real, I had all these expectations about marriage being 50 percent shared responsibilities and late-night pillow fights, but it turned out that it's extremely hard work, pretty much forever. And that's okay because I've learned to adjust my expectations, which has lowered my stress levels. So learn to let go of your expectations and set more realistic goals for yourself.

Fight or Flight System

Your body has this cool, yet complicated, system for processing dangerous stuff, like stress, to keep you safe and alive. You may know it as the "fight-or-flight" response. When something scary or stressful happens, like a man jumping in front of your car at 11 p.m., your brain sets off alarms screaming, "Danger! Danger!" A bunch of physical changes occur in your body. Your breath quickens, distributing blood faster to the body. Your muscles tense up, preparing to either freeze, get the hell out of there, or open a can of whoop-ass. To protect your vital organs, your heart rate goes up and blood moves to the center of your body.

All of this happens within seconds of that maniac jumping in front of your car. It's all good because you're prepared to deal with what's before you—although it scares the royal shite out of you. It only takes a few minutes for your body to return to normal after you make the conscious decision to swerve and avoid hitting him. That's the way the fight or flight system should work.

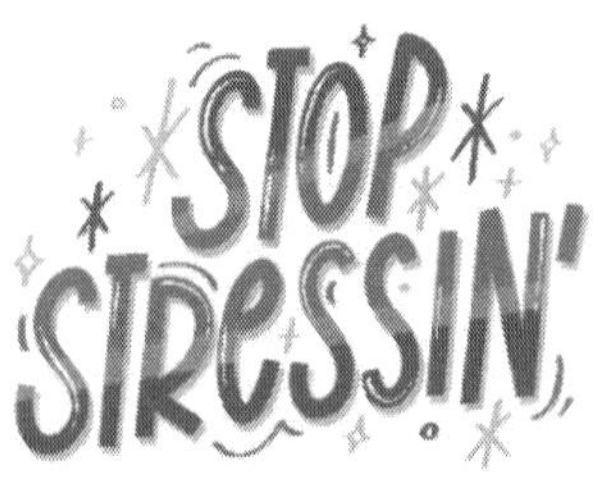

Type of Stress

This is where I tell you that not all stress is created equally, and that's a good thing. There are two types of stress, eustress and distress. Think of them as the yin and yang of stress. They are very different from each other.

Eustress, also called positive stress, is mild to moderate stress that leads to good things. Here, you see stress as a chance to learn and grow, and it pushes you to get things done. Think about moving, going to college, getting a new job, lifting weights, or raising a puppy. This is when you go through a time of major growth that leads to a positive change or a new sense of purpose, even though it is very hard. You better believe that stress was present, but it didn't serve as a negative for you. It pushed you, and you grew as a result of the stress.

This type of stress is typically short lived and brings along feelings of excitement, like the satisfaction you might feel after taking that final exam. This is because this stress is manageable, motivating, and helps you feel more resilient in the face of upcoming challenges.

On the other hand, negative stress is called distress. This is an unpleasant feeling, thought, condition, or behavior. Distress can change how you think, feel, or act, which can make it harder to deal with lupus, its symptoms, treatments, and side effects. A certain amount of distress is normal when it comes to SLE.

When stress is squeezing you, people always say the same old thing: get the hell away from stressful things. They're saying to quit that stressful job, move to a new apartment, get a new partner—like, run for the hills, girl! Stress is a threat that you must avoid at all costs.

In some situations, distress can turn into eustress. This is a nice perk. An example is when a job layoff is initially upsetting but, over time, turns into an opportunity to find a new career path. And vice versa.

Positive stress can become negative stress if it becomes too intense or lasts for too long. Just think about building a house or growing a baby if you want examples of this at play.

Stress Length Matters

How long you experience stress plays an important role in the impact it has on your health and life. The two lengths of stress we will talk about are short and long.

Short-term, yay

Short bursts of stress can be a good thing. When you lose your phone, are running late, or are cheering on the Cincinnati Bengals, you can benefit from this short-term stress. Firdaus Dhabhar, a professor at Stanford University, looked at how stress changes people both mentally and physically. He found that short-term stress gives people more energy and is an important source of fuel for the body and mind.

Research has also shown that as stress goes up, thinking skills and short-term memory improve. After this brief period of stress, the immune system grows stronger. It also helps physical wounds heal quicker, brings along more happiness and confidence, and raises your ability to get stuff done. Hooray for short-term stress for lupus peeps—bring it on!

Long-term, boo

Remember that fight or flight response? While it might come in handy when you need to dodge a predator, living in a constant state of stress is about as bad as a case of pubic lice. Basically, it's like that toxic friend you can't seem to shake. Do all you can to avoid chronic stress. It's no good for you or your SLE. Here, the length of stress extends across months and into years. Your brain gets stuck in survival mode and is on the lookout for danger even when there's no real threat to be found. Your body is already upset by the constant inflammation that lupus causes, so it is important to keep an eye on this chronic stress.

Physically

Did you know that long-term stress is linked to up to 90 percent of all illnesses and diseases?[32] It's listed as the sixth leading cause of death. Chronic stress makes you more susceptible to viral illnesses. And with lupus, this can make your disease activity worse and put you at extra risk for infections.[33] Basically, stress is the enemy of the immune system.

But that's not all—stress can also make you age faster (hello, new unwanted wrinkles!), mess with your digestion, and increase your risk of developing type 2 diabetes. And let's not forget about the impact on sex drive—stress can make you feel less frisky than a cat in a bathtub. On a more serious level, your risk of heart attack and stroke increases significantly with chronic stress.

Mentally

And it's not just physically—chronic stress can make you more likely to overeat, use drugs or alcohol, and avoid social situations. It has a negative impact on attention, memory, and managing emotions. Long-term stress can alter brain structure, especially in areas involving learning and memory.[34] It can act as a trigger for depression and anxiety.[35]

Emotionally

More people are stressed out than ever before because their emotions control their decisions and judgments without them even realizing it. Also, we do not do things that tell our bodies and nervous systems to calm down, so stress keeps coming back.

Stress Meets Spirituality

Studies point out that believing in a higher power can keep you healthy and more at peace. Attending a religious service as little as once a month has been shown to reduce the risk of death by about a third.[36] This could be because religious people are less likely to do dangerous or risky things and more likely to do healthy things like self-reflection, relaxation, and stress-relieving activities. Your spirituality can provide a sense of peace during uncertain and scary times. Remember that spirituality isn't religion based. We are all connected in this big world, and there's more than one path to your own personal nirvana, enlightenment, or heaven.

In the book *The Blue Zones*, author Dan Buettner looked into places around the world with the most people over a hundred years old to find out how they lived and what they had in common. He found that these people had a strong reason to wake up, start the day, and work toward goals, which made them live longer. Every person in the Blue Zone had their own faith. Whether they were Catholic, Adventist, Greek Orthodox, or a blend of religion and ancestor worship, it didn't matter; the point was that they all had faith in something. If you are "faithless," there's no need to join a church; instead, find a spiritual community that resonates with you and get involved there to help you deal with stress.

Stress Is Contagious

Did you know that stress is so contagious that it can be transmitted faster than the latest viral video? Whether it's a homeless person standing in the rain, a friend tripping as she walks, or a sappy commercial about dogs in need, witnessing another in pain can be stressful. The stress hormone cortisol has been found to be higher in people who witness other people completing a stressful task.[37] When someone you know suffers from a chronic illness, you might also feel extra stress. This rings true for me, as the suffering of my lupus-stricken friends has a profound effect on me. You can now see the ripple effects of your lupus battle on your entire support group.

Stress and feelings can spread in other ways, like through text messages. The receiver of an angry text will actually feel some of the sender's rage. Interesting, huh? Yale University conducted a thirty-year study on the impact of feelings in a small town in Framingham, Massachusetts. The results showed that when someone became happy or sad in this town of five thousand people, that emotion rippled throughout the entire town. Emotions, and thus stress, are contagious.

This brings to mind all of the people you choose to have in your life and the media (social media, news, movies, etc.) you consume. You better watch out, because their emotions can be caught. So, next time you encounter a stressed-out friend, don't be surprised if you suddenly start feeling the urge to scream into a pillow or eat a gallon of ice cream. Thoughtfully consider those people, activities, and news feeds that you let in.

Reflections

- There's an upside to stress, and understanding this is vital to managing its pressure and impact on both lupus and your health.

- Avoid chronic stress like the plague. It's not good for you or your SLE.
- Short-term stress gives you a boost of energy and the motivation to get stuff done.
- It's your choice to see the stress that comes your way as an opportunity for growth and meaning, even if you can't control it or don't want it.

16

Resilient AF

Character cannot be developed in ease and quiet. Only through trial and suffering can the soul be strengthened and success achieved.

—Helen Keller

It was a rough day, and my body was feeling extra cranky. I got up from my desk and reached for my mug on the kitchen island when it felt like a sandbag had been dropped on my shoulder. I dropped to my knees, yelling from the shooting pain. Oh, if only I could say this was a singular, bizarre event, but alas, it had become an unwelcome regular occurrence. A trip to the orthopedist revealed the culprit: adhesive capsulitis, or, as it's more commonly known, frozen shoulder. And, of course, because life has a flair for the dramatic, having an autoimmune disease makes you more susceptible to such delightful surprises.

Coming back from the doctor, I was sad and frustrated to have added something else to my bag of issues. I wondered when my health would plateau and softly cried while mumbling, "You got this," although it resembled more of a hesitant question than a statement.

Once home, I knew I had to have a serious heart-to-heart conversation with myself because this was the reality of my life. I had to accept and make peace with whatever came my way along this SLE quest because, clearly, it would be quite a ride. I started making a mental list of all the reasons I should be proud of myself as I thought about past problems that seemed impossible at the time but turned out to be good lessons. Whenever my mind drifted toward the dangerous territory of "Why me?" I forcefully redirected my thoughts back to the idea that I had an inner strength that could weather any storm. This internal pep rally served as a powerful reminder that life could indeed be tough and unforgiving, yet beneath it all, I remained resilient.

This frozen shoulder, the difficulties of lupus, and life's occasional hardships would not break me. Instead, they serve as reminders of the strong spirit that lives inside this chick.

This chapter takes a plunge into the world of resilience and its role in managing life's stress. We uncover practical techniques to cultivate and strengthen resilience, empowering us to face challenges head-on and bounce back from life's curveballs. As we navigate the twists and turns of life and lupus, we discover that resilience isn't just about surviving; it's about finding understanding in the chaos and using our wit as a secret weapon against stress.

The Resilience-Stress Connection

Resilience is the courage to grow from stress, and it's an often over looked resource. Studies show that people who have dealt with moderate stress in the past are better able to deal with the stress they face now.[38] Resilient people have a special way of thinking that protects them from the harmful effects of stress on their health, even when they're under immense pressure. They can navigate challenging situations without letting them take a toll on their well-being. Stress is seen as a way to grow, which shows how much resilience affects both mental health and overall health.

Embracing stress can be a powerful way to build resilience and strength. As author Kelly McGonigal says in *The Upside of Stress*, "We can transform fear into courage, isolation into connection, and suffering into meaning." The goal of life isn't to be untouched by adversity or unruffled by difficulties. It's about allowing stress to awaken courage, connection, and growth deep within you, to search for and find meaning in the suffering that stress causes, and to grow stronger from your struggles. **It's an act of bravery to find meaning in your distress.**

Resilience isn't something you're born with. These are mad skills that you can develop over time. It's about learning to take responsibility for your life and believing that you have control over your own destiny. It's about embracing the pain and discomfort of life, knowing that you can make it through and come out stronger on the other side.

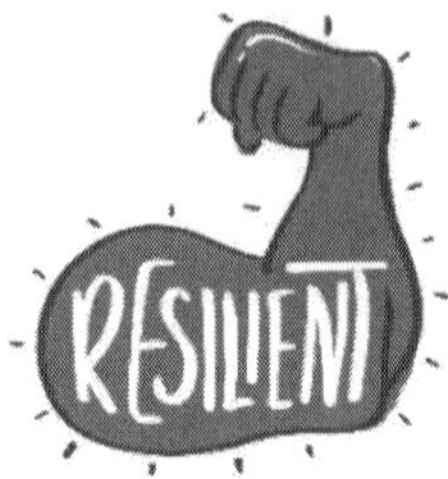

Resilience makes you stronger

When you have more resilience, you get better at not feeling bad about your SLE, stress, or whatever crap life flings your way. Knowing you have a direct impact on what happens, you are more willing to take responsibility for everything in your life. Believing that you hold the keys to your own life makes you more likely to take action to change your situation when needed.

With resilience, you're less likely to dwell on problems, feel like a victim, get far too stressed out, and turn to unhealthy ways of dealing with problems.

Resilient women are able to experience painful emotions without getting lost in them. They have core beliefs centered around having control over their lives, learning from mistakes, believing they matter in this world, and having real strengths to rely on and share with others. And their secret is that they cultivate habits that foster healthy relationships with difficult emotions.

Adopting this new mindset

Thankfully, you've got choices when it comes to seeing how stress impacts you and the resilience you tap into. You can totally shift your perspective on stress and see it as a turbocharger that gets you pumped up and ready to take on the world.

You can face stress, setbacks, and difficult emotions just like anyone else. But here's the thing: You have the power to tap into your strengths and seek support when needed. It's through resilience that you can navigate challenges, accept the situation, and adapt accordingly. By embracing it, you empower yourself to move forward, make progress, and continue on your journey toward personal growth.

Playing it safe and avoiding stress might sound safer and less scary, but it can hold you back from reaching your true potential. Yep, even the toughest situations can be like personal trainers, pushing you to grow and transform.

Remember, it's your call. You've got what it takes to overcome and thrive. You have the power to decide how you see stress and how you handle it. If you believe your vaccinations are evil, they might just turn into little monsters. You can also flip the script and see them as superhero sidekicks on your quest for better lupus health. So instead of running away from stress, give it a big bear hug. The ball's in your court, my friend.

Next time your heart is pounding from a run-in with your nemesis, think of it as your body's way of giving you the energy you need to rise to the challenge, and understand that stress is something we all deal with. The stress that comes at you is helpful. See yourself as being able to handle, learn from, and grow from the stress.

How to switch to this new way of looking at stress as a protective friend:

1. Acknowledge when you feel stressed. Notice the changes in your body. When stress arises, how does your body respond? For some, it's a racing heart or an upset stomach. Others experience headaches or sweaty hands. Take a pause and notice what you're going through.
2. Welcome the stress. Think back to the definition of stress, which is what arises when something you care about is at stake. Do you really give a flying fuck about this stress? Yeah? Okay, why does it matter to you? This awareness will allow you to respond more appropriately to the stress by either preparing for battle or letting it go.
3. Use the energy and motivation that come from stress to do something and take action. Don't waste it trying to control or manage the stress. The question is, "What can you do right now to manage this stress?"

Careful What You Believe

A 1993 study found that people who were highly stressed out and believed stress was harmful had a whopping 43 percent increased risk of dying early.[39] But get this, those who had high stress but saw stress as a good thing had the lowest overall risk of dying. So, it's not just stress itself that's the problem; it's the combo of stress and thinking it's a health hazard that can be deadly.

You better check yourself before you wreck yourself when it comes to your view of stress.

Boost That Resilience

If you want to be more resilient, you can build up your physical, emotional, and mental reserves. That way, when stress comes knocking, you'll be ready to handle it without breaking too much of a sweat. These strategies include focusing on your strengths, having a purpose, volunteering, and accepting what life brings.

Grow your strengths

Let's talk about strength, shall we? Put your energy into growing what you're good at—the things you do well. Here's the thing: What you consider to be your strengths is not always consistent with how you actually behave, as studies have shown. That means you might actually be the least qualified person to provide information about what you're awesome at. For help in determining where you rock, ask three people who know you well what your strengths are, and focus on those bad boys.

To boost resilience, tap into those strengths. Notice that I didn't say to strengthen what you're bad at, and I know that's a bit weird because most people would say to do this to be "well-rounded." Don't focus on your weaknesses. That's a trap! When you focus on building up your weaknesses, you typically let go of the things you're stellar at.

Sense of purpose

When the world feels scary and your health becomes uncertain, having a sense of purpose can ground you. Your life's purpose refers to the fundamental driving forces that shape and dictate why you get out of bed in the morning. This purpose can help steer important decisions, influence your behavior, provide a sense of direction, and inject some meaning into your life. When you have a lot of important, fun, and exciting things going on in your life, it's much easier to stay focused and not let the bad things get in the way.

Don't worry, your purpose doesn't have to be something huge like removing all guns from the world. It can be something as simple as being kind or helping out in your community.

Share the care

Speaking of community, why not share love and care for others? Surely, we could all use more of this! By doing kind things for people, you'll feel better, and your stress levels will drop. It's a win-win situation, as caring creates resilience. By doing concrete things that contribute to the greater good at large, you can change your outlook, be calmer, and feel better. This can be done by cleaning up a park, telling your fourth-grade teacher she was the best, or paying for a stranger's coffee.

When people are having a hard time, they help others because it's in their nature to do so. Studies show that people are kinder and more generous after a traumatic event like a hurricane or earthquake. Even when we are in pain, we have a strong desire to help others. This is why people with chronic pain who become peer mentors or give back to others feel less pain and have deeper life meaning.

Build up relationships

Developing stronger friendships is like building social armor that protects you from stress monsters. We humans are social creatures who need others to thrive, and investing time in friendships can bring you all the warm and fuzzy feelings. It's like a happiness exchange program—invest a little, get a lot back. Diversifying your friendships is like creating a personal fan club that cheers you on through thick and thin.

And if you're already in a friendship, spend more time together than you do on social media. The best part? It only takes thirty hours to form a casual friendship, but three hundred hours to reach BFF status. This means start scheduling those coffee dates or walking meetups, and don't forget to reach out to your pals when you're feeling down in the dumps.

Accept reality

As humans, we naturally want to avoid pain, emotional pain included. I mean, who wants to feel like a soggy tissue when you can feel like a fluffy cloud? But our defense mechanisms can be sneaky, like trying to hide a fart in an elevator. Denial is the big bad wolf of defense mechanisms—it may feel good at first, but it only makes you more fragile in the long run. Resilient people are like superheroes who embrace short-term pain for long-term gain. When you accept the reality of a situation, you can endure discomfort like a boss and emerge stronger on the other side. Embrace your feelings, accept reality, and build up that warrior spirit within you.

Reflections

- Resilient women have unique mindsets that protect them from stress and allow them to navigate challenges without compromising their well-being.
- Embracing stress as an opportunity for growth builds resilience and strength.
- Resilience is a skill that can be developed over time by taking responsibility for your life and believing in your ability to control your destiny.
- Boost resilience by focusing on strengths, finding purpose, caring for others, and developing strong relationships.

17

Let's Be Mindful, Shall We?

Living in the moment, it's a gift. That's why they call it the present.

—Ted Lasso

Mindfulness has taught me to be more present in this one life I've been given and better manage what comes my way, but it wasn't always like this.

I was a lab rat for mindfulness when I enrolled in a six-week clinical trial. I participated in weekly classes on how to be mindful, and I was required to sit still daily and practice what I learned for thirty to sixty minutes. Since this whole mindfulness thing was new to me, it was hard to maintain my focus in the beginning because my mind zipped from one thought to another. "For the love of all things peaceful, just be quiet for a second, will ya?" I begged my brain.

Something happened after a few weeks of practicing. I began to get into this mindfulness groove. The process of following my thoughts became a bit easier. I could notice that I was telling myself stories in my head, then redirect myself back to my breath. One day, I remember thinking that I could live a life completely present in the moment. How very Zen of me!

A full-day silent retreat marked the end of the trial, and it was shockingly lovely, as I had never gone a day without talking in my life.

Finally, I was off the hook. I was free to be completely absorbed in my thoughts again. Whoopee.

And I did just this until I got my first autoimmune diagnosis. Then, my health demanded that I take stock of what was important. It seemed that living a distracted life didn't mesh well with a body fighting constant inflammation. The more I tried to ignore and push through, the worse I felt. Then I remembered back to my time in the trial, all the hours I spent being mindful, and all the benefits it offered. I figured it couldn't hurt to give it a try again.

Slowly, I put it into my daily routine. I carved out time to follow my breath in and out. I drank tea in the morning and worked on being fully present. I turned off my radio in the car, drove in silence, and tried not to get lost in my thoughts. Eventually, my body and mind responded positively. I felt less stressed, my mind felt more centered, and I was less bothered by people and situations.

Being a "lab rat" for mindfulness seems to have given me the gift of being in the moment, and it came just when I needed it.

Whether you're new to the idea of mindfulness or looking to enhance your practice, this chapter has got you covered. Discover why mindfulness is so important (and worth all the hype), learn about the amazing ways it can positively impact your body, and find out just how simple it is to incorporate into your daily life. Get ready for an accessible and transformative journey!

Life on Autopilot

Have you ever magically arrived at work without realizing you were driving there? Research reveals that nearly half of our lives are spent in a state of mind-wandering, dwelling on the past or future instead of being in the moment. Living a life on autopilot may seem harmless for simple tasks, like folding laundry and watching YouTube, but it can have more significant consequences when the stakes are higher.

Fortunately, there is a remedy—mindfulness. Here, we can untangle ourselves from the constant mental chatter and feel more present in this one life we've been given.

What's the Point of Mindfulness?

Mindfulness is a state of awareness. A focus on the present moment. As Dan Harris describes in *Meditation for Fidgety Skeptics*, it's the ability to observe the happenings within your mind without getting caught up in them. Mindfulness can be done in different ways, but the goal of all of them is to reach a state of alert, focused relaxation by paying attention to thoughts and feelings without judging them.

At its core, mindfulness involves paying attention to what comes up in your mind, throughout your body, and in the world around you. It frees you from constant mental spirals and brings you back to the here and now. It teaches you to stop letting your thoughts run your life and instead simply observe them.

When you begin to pay attention to your mind, you'll notice just how noisy it is. Holy crap! You'll be surprised that it never shuts up. You're wondering what to eat for dinner, when that book will arrive from Amazon, and how long the neighbor's kid can actually scream before he loses his voice (the answer to this is a long forty-eight minutes).

This is where the power of mindfulness comes in. You'll begin to separate yourself from your thoughts by drawing a wee bit of space between the two and not always jumping from one thought directly onto another. The goal isn't to turn off your brain (as if you could), but to let go of thoughts as they arise. It isn't about blocking out negative thoughts or stress, but rather recognizing them while knowing that you don't have to react to them. Simple practices like counting your breaths or repeating a calming phrase like "relax" can help achieve this.

Quick note: Mindfulness is not based on a particular religion. Prayer is when you speak to your higher source. Mindfulness is when you listen.

The Lupus Link

Now, when it comes to your health, **what messes with your well-being also messes with your lupus.** Your brain is like a danger-detecting missile, always on the lookout for trouble. But here's the thing: having a brain that's constantly buzzing is not great for your health. Chronic stress from this nonstop activity leads to more inflammation, which is as bad as deep-fried Oreos at the county fair.

That's where mindfulness swoops in to save the day. By reducing chronic stress, it protects your body and mind from the harmful effects of prolonged stress. You are creating space in your mind by figuring out what is essential and prioritizing it, resulting in a deeper sense of calm, reconnecting with your body, and feeling like a superhero with better health.

But don't think of mindfulness like celery juice, where it's supposed to miraculously heal everything, because it won't. It is not a cure-all for everything, especially not for lupus. It's more like a trusty sidekick that equips you with awesome tools to handle the ongoing stress you face. It can ease symptoms and give your overall health a power-up.

Easy-Peasy Mindfulness

Mindfulness can be broken into three easy steps, but don't underestimate something that appears simple because you still have to actually do it. That's where something easy becomes a challenge. The process is as follows:

Step 1: Be aware when your mind has wandered and/or you're lost in your thoughts.

Step 2: Notice what you're thinking, and let go of these ideas.

Step 3: Take a breath in and out.

Mindfulness is a skill, just like taking the perfect profile pic or finding the juiciest watermelon (why is this so hard?). As a result, it takes a dedicated effort to cultivate a new habit, which means you need to set aside time to practice each day.

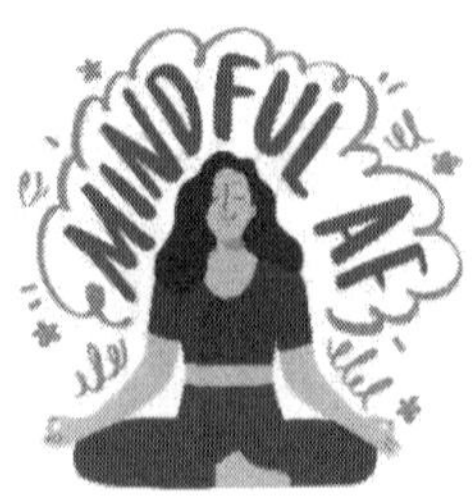

Powerful Benefits

When I asked my rheumatologist what she thought was the most important thing for a woman with lupus to do for her health that was in her control, she said mindfulness. That speaks volumes to me. See, mindfulness is powerful and totally worth it—even my rheumatologist agrees.

Now, wait until you hear all of the clinically proven benefits you can get just by simply noticing that you're thinking and following your breath. You'll be shocked. What you get out of this is much more than the work you have to put into it.

Regularly practicing mindfulness can offer up a lot of incredible mental and physical benefits:

- You'll strengthen your immune system and lower your blood pressure, heart rate, and inflammation.[40]
- Your sleep will improve.
- The cells in your body actually age slower.
- Chronic pain will be reduced by up to 57 percent.[41]
- You'll be better able to manage anxiety and depression without drugs.[42]
- You'll protect your body and mind from the harmful effects of prolonged stress.[43]
- You'll have improved focus, memory, and logic.
- You'll have the ability to be compassionate and forgiving of your own mistakes and others'.
- Your relationships will improve and you'll have fewer conflicts.
- You'll build deeper reserves of physical well-being, mental clarity, emotional balance, and resilience.

Mindfulness Is the Mental Gym

By repeatedly bringing your attention back to the breath each time it wanders off, concentration builds and deepens, much as muscles develop by repetitively lifting weights.

—Jon Kabat-Zinn

Mindfulness has five main ideas that work together like a mental gym to make the brain stronger.

Nonjudgmental: Here you learn to not believe everything your mind thinks. You observe your thoughts without judgment. Instead of labeling them as good or bad, you recognize that not everything your mind thinks is true or accurate.

Self-Awareness: Mindfulness allows you to gain a deeper understanding of your thoughts, patterns, and behaviors. My therapist likes to remind me that the majority of people are lacking in this department, but not you. Oh no, you're going to do better. By peering into your mind, you strive to see reality as it is without trying to change or resist it.

Acceptance: This develops from allowing your current situation to be just as it is without wishing things were different. Acceptance involves working with what you have instead of pushing against it. It helps you believe in yourself and your ability to handle problems, even ones that are caused by lupus.

Self-Compassion: Being mindful helps you be kind to yourself. It involves being an internal, loving, and encouraging friend rather than a harsh critic when you are going through a tough time. Self-compassion means that you know it is okay to make mistakes and that you are valuable. It's saying, "I'm a badass even when I screw up."

Non-Striving: Instead of looking for change all the time, non-striving asks you to be in the moment and accept it. It teaches you to be patient and trust how life unfolds. This lets you be who you are without rushing or forcing things to happen.

Adding More Mindfulness to Your Life

If you want to dip your toe into the pool of mindfulness, you don't have to worry about having to give up a lot of time or space to do this. All you need is a few minutes, a little bit of focus, and maybe an app (if you want).

Length

I bet you are wondering, "Hmm, how long do I really need to do this mindfulness thing?" In the beginning, set a goal of practicing for three to five minutes. But please know that even one mindful breath can offer a benefit. If this works well, practice for a longer time and consider two short sessions versus one long one.

Frequency

Consistency is key here, meaning a brief practice each day is better than a long session once a week. The reason is that the more you invest, the more you can get out of it.

When

Figure out what time of day makes the most sense for you to practice. While mindfulness can be practiced any time of the day, it's easier for some in the morning, when the mind is quieter and more refreshed.

Where

A cool thing about mindfulness is that it can be done anytime, anywhere, except when you're asleep. As a newbie, it's far easier to begin practicing in a quiet spot with no distractions. Once you're comfortable here, you can progress to noisier places. Then put these skills on full display at Thanksgiving as you breathe your way through the meal despite your grandma suggesting you need a new haircut. Mindfulness can also be done before you respond to an email, in a conversation, or while eating lunch.

Apps

You don't need much to practice mindfulness, but apps can help. I use a free one called Mindfulness Bell. This simple app makes a ding noise every thirty minutes during the workday, and it snaps me out of my fog and back into the present moment. Other apps, like Calm and Headspace, offer great practice resources too, with guided mindfulness sessions across a variety of topics. They even have sessions on pain and sleep. Give a few a try to see if they help you practice. Some insurance companies offer these apps at a low cost or for free to their policyholders.

Mindfulness Methods That Work for You

Get rid of the idea that mindfulness can only be practiced sitting cross-legged and chanting "om" on repeat. **There is no one "right way" to practice mindfulness.**

Paying attention to your breathing is one of the most common ways to develop this, but there are many other ways, such as focusing on your body or the sounds around you. These techniques help develop steady, present-moment attention. Mindfulness can be formally or informally incorporated into your life. Here are some suggestions to find a way that works best for you:

1. **Walking:** When you walk, feel your feet hit the ground with each step and pay attention to the sensation in your body. For others who don't use their feet to move around, this can also be mindful moving, where you focus on what you feel and notice as you move in a wheelchair or other device.
2. **Sensory-guided:** This means paying close attention to what you hear, feel, smell, taste, and/or see. Sitting outside and feeling the breeze on your skin or listening to the sounds around you are both good ways to do this.
3. **Body scan:** Slowly and on purpose, move your mind from the top of your head to the tips of your toes while you follow your breath. The focus is on being calm and aware while keeping a link between what you feel and how your body feels. If you're in pain, notice the feeling without trying to block it, as you get more at ease with the unpleasant feelings.
4. **Waiting:** When you find yourself waiting—at the store, in traffic, for a meeting to start—don't pick up your phone. Focus on what's around you. Hear the sounds, see the sights, and enjoy the sense of aliveness.
5. **Eating:** Instead of eating in front of a phone or TV, eat with no distractions, close your eyes, and savor the taste of a strawberry. The goal is to notice the food while your brain rests.
6. **Showering:** Notice as the water hits your body, the smell of the soap, and the spray of the water around you. Feel your hands touch your body and be present.

For me, I'm more of an informal practitioner. I like to do this daily when walking my dog, Mobey. I leave my phone at home and pay attention to the nature around me. Finally, when feeling extra stressed or in pain, I go back to a formal practice by sitting in a chair and following my breath.

Reflections

- Mindfulness is as good for your body and mind as it is for lupus.
- Accept that this will take time to learn while you find the method that works best for you.

- Be patient and kind to yourself in the process of integrating mindfulness into your life.
- Let go of expectations for yourself and how this "should" work, and just practice.

18

Just Breathe

Breathe, darling. This is just a chapter.
It's not your whole story.

—S.C. Lourie

I've been through an MRI before, but this time felt like I was being stuffed into that tube like a tightly packed sausage. Picture this: a snug KN95 facemask with a metal shield on top, and then entering the MRI machine with its symphony of sounds that made me question if I accidentally signed up for a wild heavy metal concert instead. I kept repeating, "It's fine, it's fine," but deep down, I knew I wasn't. Claustrophobia and fear washed over me, but there was no escape. I was trapped. It was like a one-way ticket to an anxiety attack. Internally, I was screaming, "Get me the hell out of here!" Externally, my breath quickened, and sweat dripped down my face, pooling inside my facemask.

Thankfully, I had a secret weapon up my sleeve—a decade of practicing breathwork. It was the only thing that kept me from losing my shit that day. I mustered all my strength and slowed down my breathing, expanding my lungs with each inhale of four and exhaling for a count of eight. My breathing rhythm helped me gradually calm down and clear my mind. It was my lifeline amidst the claustrophobic chaos, and I was so grateful that I could tap into it when it was really needed.

Regular attention to your breath can save you from a breakdown, like it did for me. It can also help lower stress and offer a bunch of good benefits for your lupus body. This chapter will teach you about the importance of your breath and how it helps with mindfulness. You'll learn ways to incorporate breathing tips and techniques that help you feel better, and you'll see why humming "Happy Birthday" is good for you too.

Vital Breathing

Stop what you are doing and take a deep breath. Now let it out. Feel better? Good, read on.

You can live for weeks without food and several hours without water. But you'd survive only a few minutes without air—don't you believe me? Go ahead, give it a try. Even though we take twenty-five thousand breaths each day, it is rarely considered in the equation of health.

But it should be, as breathing affects every part of your body, including stress levels, blood pressure, and heart rate. Learning how to control your breathing can influence your energy, focus, choices, and how you feel in the moment. In *Breath*, James Nestor writes, "No matter what we eat, how much we exercise, how resilient our genes are, or how skinny, young, or wise we are, none of it matters unless we're breathing correctly. **The missing pillar of health is breath.**" Your breathing impacts both your lupus and how it's managed. All in all, that breath of yours is pretty damn essential.

You might as well use breathing to your advantage since it is a human necessity.

What Is Breathwork?

Breathwork is a wide range of breathing exercises and techniques used to control breathing, from deep breathing to belly breathing and more. It can involve taking a deep breath before getting a shot or slowing down a racing heart after an accident. If you can believe it, there are as many ways to breathe as there are foods to eat. Chew on that idea.

The power of deep, cleansing breaths is well known—it powers down our stress responses and helps us feel more grounded. Your ability to breathe in different ways can have a huge effect on your physical, mental, emotional, and spiritual health. If it helps your body, it can help your lupus.

Besties: Breathwork and Mindfulness

Breathwork and mindfulness are dynamic duos that amplify each other's superpowers. Picture this: mindfulness is the calm, observant guru, and breathwork is the trusty sidekick that keeps everything in rhythm.

Both are wonderful practices that offer shared and unique benefits, but they definitely have their differences. Overall, mindfulness is great at getting yourself to live in the present moment, while breathwork focuses on consciously regulating and deepening the breath.

If you struggle to sit down and concentrate on your thoughts, using breathwork is a great alternative to traditional mindfulness, and your body and mind will benefit too.

Breathing Is a Lost Art

Did you know that your typical way of breathing is probably messing up your body and its functions in a lot of different ways? Yup. You may be sabotaging your health without realizing it, and that includes your mood, digestion, nervous system, and ability to sleep. Yikes!

As a species, 80 percent of us have lost the ability to breathe correctly, with grave consequences. With the impact of lupus already weighing heavily on you, breathing correctly is more important than ever. As babies, we breathe perfectly, but we pick up bad habits as we age. Some ways it can show up are with over-breathing, chest breathing, or unintentionally holding your breath, like when you're on a roller coaster.

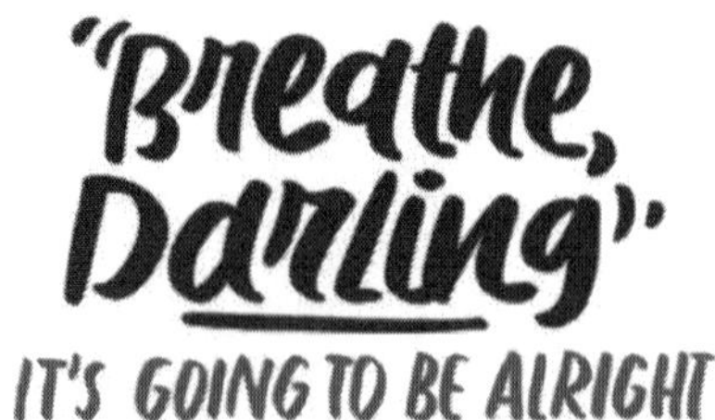

Good Breathwork

Optimizing how you breathe is very important, especially since you have lupus. Luckily, doing this isn't all that complicated. If you want to improve your health and alleviate pain, stress, and tension, all you have to do is adopt some simple breathing ideas.[44]

Seal those lips

Are you a mouth breather? Do you sleep with your mouth open, snore, or have an itchy nose? Your answer is super important, so you better be sure.

Mouth breathing is not great for you—in fact, it's really bad. Small problems, like the changing mouth bacteria that increases the risk for cavities and gum disease. Medium-sized problems, like chronic allergies and recurring sinus infections, show up. And then there are big, huge problems like the increased risk of sleep apnea and asthma from the lower amount of oxygen that comes from mouth breathing.

Think of your nose as a factory that filters and refines the air for your body while heating and pressurizing it. It also makes the air more humid, which is better for the lungs. Nestor found that breathing through your nose makes your body release different hormones, affecting everything from your menstrual cycle to your anxiety level and more. It can even help with your fitness routine. Ain't this body grand?

Breathing through your nose greatly increases the body's nitric oxide levels and boosts the lungs' ability to absorb oxygen. This isn't the laughing gas you get from your dentist's office; it occurs naturally. You will have more energy throughout the day as nitric oxide increases blood circulation. Plus, nitric oxide is pretty cool as it's antifungal, antiviral, antiparasitic, and antibacterial, leaving the immune system stronger to fight infections.

Every time you take a breath, make sure it goes in and out through that nose of yours and not your mouth, even when you're exercising or sleeping.

Belly breathing

Belly breathing is one of the simplest forms of breathwork; it's arguably the easiest to do and can be practiced whenever and wherever. This type of breathing is typically done to relieve stress and correct breathing patterns, among plenty of other benefits. It's not just about getting a bunch of air in. Rather, it's about using the right muscles and the right breath rhythm to tell the body to relax.

Belly breathing has long been used in tai chi, mindfulness practices, and yoga. It is when you intentionally breathe slowly and deeply through your nose while keeping your chest as still as possible.

Here's how to practice belly breathing:

- Get into a comfortable position. You can choose to sit, lie down, or stand.
- Place one hand on your chest and the other on your stomach.
- Take a deep breath, feeling your stomach push against your hand.
- Slowly exhale, noticing the way your stomach lowers. Try to keep your chest still throughout the exercise.
- Continue to inhale and exhale this way for as long as you want.

Slow it down

Did you know that the animals who live the longest breathe the least? Think about it, a turtle can live to be three hundred years old and take only four breaths per minute. Whales take a single breath a minute and live a hundred years or more. Dogs, on the other hand, take around thirty breaths a minute, and mice take 80 to 230, explaining why their lifespan is pretty darn short. The average adult takes twelve to twenty breaths per minute.

The perfect slow breath is an inhale of 5.5 seconds and then an exhale of 5.5 seconds through the nose. This is about 5.5 breaths a minute. By taking deeper, slower breaths, your lungs can relish in the extra oxygen, lower pain, and live longer.

If you want to try this out, use a timer to practice. Stretch your inhales and exhales out to five to six seconds each through the nose. Or you can slowly count from 1 to 6 as your breath cycles. I've found the free app called iBreathe helpful for practicing this.

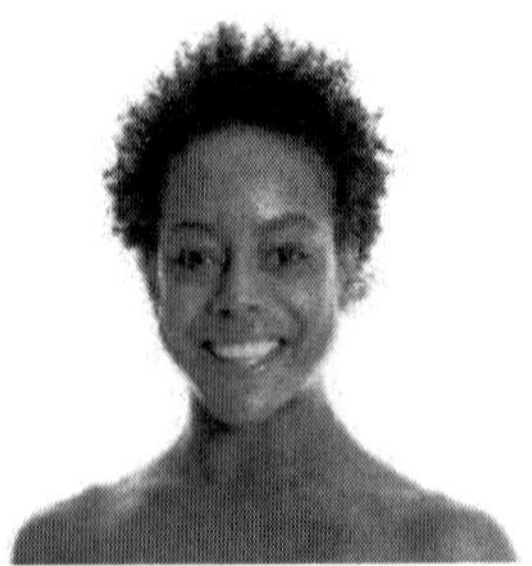

Lupus Warrior Profile

Victoria Gibbs (@whatgibbs) is an inspiring NYC woman who effortlessly blends her roles as an ultra-flexible yogi and a passionate lupus advocate. Her quest unfolds through her career as a dancer, where Victoria developed a profound understanding of the intricate link between daily habits and their impact on the body. From recognizing the value of ample sleep to emphasizing the importance of hydration, Victoria's insights illuminate the path to mindful living with lupus. She urges women with lupus to develop a deep sense of awareness and be aware of the daily fluctuations of the mind and body. Victoria's unwavering commitment to these principles became a lifeline during her battle with an aortic aneurysm, proving the transformative power of her mindful approach. Her resounding message is, "Keep showing up. Be willing to try," and this serves as a powerful reminder to break free from self-imposed limitations and remain open to the countless possibilities that surround you.

Chill out with long exhales

Put your hand over your heart. Take a slow, long breath. You should feel your heart rate speed up. When you let that breath out, your heart slows down. Exhaling activates your parasympathetic system. This is the system that helps control your body's response during times of rest and lowers your heart rate and blood pressure.

With slow, long exhales, your body will become calmer and more relaxed, telling your brain that all is well inside. This step will help you get out of a state of chronic stress and change your attitude for the better by lowering your anxiety.

Below is my favorite easy breathing exercise, which I cannot recommend enough. When the plane is bumpy and I think, "OMG, the plane is going down," I use this technique. It helps me regain my composure and de-stress. Use this whenever you feel nervous, angry, or scared.

- Breathe in for a count of four.
- Breathe out for a count of eight, or until you feel your lungs squeezing out all the air.
- Repeat until your heart rate, nerves, and breathing have chilled out.

When in Doubt, Hum It Out

Instead of reaching for coffee or caffeine when you're feeling tired, get a giant boost of energy from nitric oxide by humming. Practice this by humming the song "Happy Birthday," taking a deep breath in, and making a slow, steady hum when you let that breath go. Besides tickling your nose and teeth, you'll notice that this is that perfect breath coming into play.

How to do this humdinger:

1. Pick a private place, or else people will think you've gone crazy.
2. Take a slow breath through your nose.
3. Very slowly exhale while humming until there's nothing left in your lungs.
4. Recover with a deep inhale, then hum it out again.

Reflections

- Breathwork is a technique used to control breathing and boost health.
- A slow exhale helps you calm your nerves and chill out.
- Breathe in and out of your nose whenever possible.
- Hum it out to get more energy.

19

Transforming Lupus, One Bite at a Time

You are what you eat, so don't be fast, cheap, easy, or fake.

—Unknown

After my lupus diagnosis, I became fixated on nutrition, experimenting with every meal plan imaginable, from Mediterranean to vegan. I even sought guidance from a celebrity trainer who poo-pooed anything that wasn't non-GMO or organic. She made healthy eating seem like a full-time job. Talk about high maintenance.

But here's the kicker: all this excessive scrutiny just left me completely stuck. I had no idea what to eat anymore and often skipped meals altogether—definitely not a good approach. Looking back, I realize I was taking it way too seriously and going overboard.

I got help figuring out what to eat by working closely with a registered dietitian to solve my food problems. Together, we came up with ways to improve my diet with healthy fats and lots of veggies and set a goal of keeping my daily sugar intake to twenty grams or less. It felt like I was giving up sugar entirely, but it made a world of difference and kept me satisfied.

Gradually, I came to understand that nourishing food held the key to feeling good. Finding the right way to eat for my lupus is important, but it doesn't have to be a never-ending quest for the holy grail of nutrition. Just like breathing properly, nutrition is only one part of how healthy we are as a whole. Lesson learned: Sometimes it's better to let go of the magnifying glass and just grab a sandwich, even if that's on non-organic bread.

Food is one thing we have control over, and so much weight is placed on its influence. Yes, nutrition plays an important part in your overall lupus saga, but you do not have to be on a diet, starving yourself, and getting all hangry just for SLE. In fact, remove the word diet from your mind and replace it with the concept that good nutrition helps make lupus more manageable. This chapter will provide essential information and the resources to make healthy choices for your body and your disease. Upgrading your nutrition can have a significant impact on your lupus and is a vital piece of your treatment plan. Put down that fancy organic granola bar and read on.

Eating Right with Lupus

"Drink hot lemon water in the morning. Only eat wild salmon. Kale is the best," blah, blah, blah. There are so many rules about how and what we should eat. It's enough to make you not want to snarf down a bag of hot Cheetos and get a flaming butthole in return. It's not surprising that 80 percent of Americans are totally conflicted about what to eat.[45] It feels like the wild west out there for nutrition, and there's an overwhelming amount of information to sort through to find out what's really best.

This situation is made even harder with lupus in the mix. Since the root of lupus is chronic inflammation, it makes sense to pay particular attention to using food as a way to better manage your disease and tamp down flares.

Best Lupus "Diet" Plan

There is a hot debate about the best diet plan when it comes to lupus. Paleo, keto, gluten-free, anti-inflammatory, Mediterranean, and the DASH diet have all been thrown around as possible contenders to win this award.

Take a slow breath here; the winner is . . . none of them! According to the National Institute of Arthritis and Musculoskeletal and Skin Diseases, no research has proven that a specific diet helps with lupus symptoms. Also, **there are no foods that are known to cause or cure lupus**. Licensed dietitian Tanya Freirich, known as The Lupus Dietitian online, says that patients with lupus can find success with a wide range of dietary approaches. Because of differences in genetics, lupus symptoms, lifestyle, and personal preference, what food choices help one person with lupus may not help another with lupus.

Now that you know there are no magic foods or diets, you might be wondering what you should eat. The best options to reduce inflammation and help with flares are to eat more fresh food and less foods with a lot of sugar, trans-fat, and processed foods. This isn't surprising to hear, is it? Most people, no matter what diseases they have, are told to eat this way.

Not only can lupus be better managed with your diet, but your overall lupus experience can also improve.

Personalized Approach

As much as I'd love to tell you to go gluten-free or something like this (because it's so much easier to know exactly what to do), it's not happening. There are no "exacts" for lupus, as you know, because every woman has a unique relationship with this disease. This also means that there isn't one specific way to use nutrition to best manage your symptoms. It takes trial and error, tracking of symptoms, and close observation to see how your body responds to what you feed it. The challenge is for you to figure out what's best for you and find ways to eat like this consistently across a lifetime.

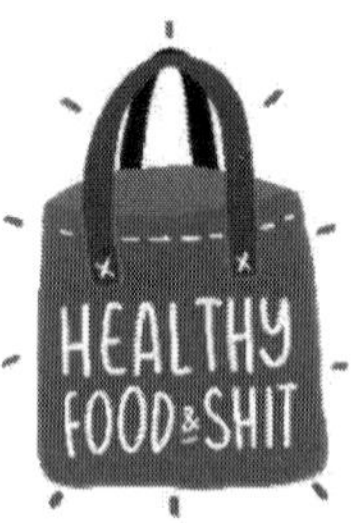

Nuts and Legumes

Lupus can be better controlled with a diet where legumes and nuts are central.[46] When people with lupus ate nuts and legumes, their symptoms went down by 41 percent.[47]

Because they have good fats and nutrients, nuts can help the immune system. Sunflower seeds and almonds are two that stand out due to their higher amounts of vitamin E. Grab a handful of nuts in place of those cookies and snack happily. Be aware of how much you eat here because those lil' nuts can pack a powerful punch of calories.

What's a legume? Think of beans, chickpeas, lentils, and peanuts—they are incredibly cheap and rich in micronutrients, protein, and healthy fat sources. These foods keep you full for longer and are a staple in the Mediterranean diet.

Eat More Plants

Surprisingly, only 9 percent of adults eat the recommended amount of daily produce. The government suggests a minimum of 1.5 to two cups of fruit and two to three cups of vegetables daily. Even though they have so many positive effects on health, it seems that few people actually eat enough.

The largest nutrition study ever published, known as EPIC, investigated the link between diet, cancer, chronic diseases, lifestyle, and environmental factors across fifteen years. The results showed that eating more fruits and vegetables lowered the risk of dying early from any cause. Scientists determined that a woman could expect to live fourteen years longer if she ate at least five servings of fruits and vegetables every day, didn't smoke, worked out consistently, and drank in moderation.[48]

Plants reduce inflammation, make the immune system stronger, and lower your risk for cancer. In a 2022 study, patients with lupus who ate more vegetables had less joint and muscle pain. It also helped with their mood, fatigue, and weight management.[49]

If you're needing to add in more veggies and fruit like I do, registered dietitian Kristen Norton offers up the following produce tips:

- At the grocery, take several laps around the produce section. With extra time here, your eyes will be open to new possibilities in variety and color. From this tip, I had my first chayote (light-green squash from Mexico) salad recently, and it tasted like a mix between a zucchini and a cucumber. Yummy.
- Fresh produce is great, but so are canned and frozen versions. These are still chocked full of nutrients and fiber, and they can save you money. Sometimes canned is better too, like how tomatoes have increased antioxidants after being heated.
- The crisper drawer in the fridge isn't offering perks for your produce. Instead, store them at eye level, where you'll be more tempted to nosh on them.

- As soon as you buy veggies, wash them and store them in containers. This makes it more convenient, and it's more likely that you'll actually eat them.
- Grate zucchini and carrots to place into sauces and baked goods, like muffins.

Eat More of This

It is time to dish on the nutritious foods that are also lupus friendly. Frei rich recommends prioritizing eating more of the foods listed below:

Green and white tea are especially good for you because they have powerful antioxidants and other nutrients that lower the risk of cognitive decline. Buy high quality tea and learn how to brew it correctly to maximize its health benefits.

Ginger's anti-inflammatory and antioxidant properties make your immune system stronger, lower blood sugar, and help your body digest food. Chop this up for a stir fry or add it to a drink with honey to soothe an upset belly or congested head.

Turmeric is a powerful spice and natural antioxidant that contains curcumin. Curcumin may help reduce inflammation and help manage inflammatory conditions, according to some promising research.[50] You can either use this heavily as a spice in your food or consider taking it as a capsule along with black pepper, as it helps with absorption. It is unsafe to use during pregnancy.

Cinnamon isn't just good for your morning oatmeal; it's also a nice source of fiber, vitamin K, iron, manganese, and calcium. The flavonoid compounds found in cinnamon are good at fighting both chronic and acute inflammation.

Quercetin-rich foods are powerful antioxidants to add to your diet. Apples, onions, green and black tea, red wine, blueberries, and broccoli are foods heavy in these sources.

Omega-3 fatty acids may show promise for symptom management in the treatment of SLE.[51] Ideally, omega-3 fatty acids are typically found in oily fish like salmon and sardines, walnuts, flaxseed, chia seeds, and hemp seeds. Overall, it's wise to avoid fish with high mercury levels.

With more antioxidants than blueberries and more fiber than oatmeal, flax, hemp, and chia seeds help heal the digestive tract and are high in omega-3. I put all three of these in my oatmeal in the morning.

Watch out list

Now onto the foods to watch out for or stay away from altogether:

Avoid **alfalfa sprouts** and **mung bean sprouts** because they boost the immune system, and you seriously don't need more of this.

Any **immune-boosting supplement** is a no-no. Your immune system is quite active already—too much so. Go ahead and throw out that echinacea, spirulina, and vitamin E. With vitamin C, it really depends, says nutritionist Freirich. She suggests getting vitamin C from foods and not worrying about taking mega doses of supplements. It's not great to consume so much if you have kidney damage as well.

Highly processed foods like chips, cookies, and beloved Fritos need to go bye-bye. So tasty with the high salt and sugar added in, but so bad for you and highly addictive. These simple carbohydrates are often lacking in nutrients like fiber and vitamins. Just a heads up: processed foods can be pretty sneaky with their trans-fat content. They often contain partially hydrogenated oils, which can increase your risk for heart disease. So, if you're looking out for your health, it's probably best to steer clear of those types of foods.

Limit your daily intake of **sugar**, as it fuels inflammation and is in just about everything, from bread to BBQ sauce. The American Heart Association recommends twenty-six grams of sugar a day, while the average American eats a whopping seventy-seven grams. Drinks account for the majority of this sugar. And let's be real, those sugary treats are only making your SLE symptoms worse. Know that those artificial sugars are not a good replacement for the real thing either because they negatively affect your gut bacteria.

Nitrates are a preservative and can be commonly found in deli meat, ham, sausage, and hotdogs. It's a good idea to limit how much of these you eat. Sure, there are also nitrates that naturally occur in vegetables, fruits, and some herbs, and those are just fine.

Speaking of meat, watch your protein levels. A high-protein diet is especially unhealthy for people with lupus-related kidney diseases.[52]

While they don't have to be avoided, take a close look at how your body responds to garlic, dairy, and alcohol. These foods can act as triggers and cause inflammation to worsen for some. Figure out how each one of these affects you.

Reflections

- There's no one way to eat best for lupus or a magical food that'll remove your SLE.
- Keep caring about what you eat because it matters.
- Work hard to get more plants, nuts, and legumes into your daily diet.
- Limit sugar, processed foods, and nitrates, and avoid alfalfa sprouts and mung bean sprouts.

20

From Kale to Cake: The Epic Quest for a Balanced Diet

Moderation. Small helpings. Sample a little bit of everything. These are the secrets of happiness and good health.

—Julia Child

My approach to nutrition today is vastly different from the past. I do my best to make the right decisions for my body and lupus. Sure, it's not always easy, and there are times when temptations come on strong and my taste buds have a mind of their own. It's a constant battle to resist the siren call of French fries and ice cream and embrace my inner "normal" American.

But then I remind myself of all the incredible benefits that come with good nutrition. I picture my body as this amazing vessel, and I owe it to myself to treat it right. So I put on my healthy decision-making cape and make choices based on what's best for me, even if it means passing on that extra slice of cake or swapping quinoa for white rice.

I'm committed to this path as long as I'm alive, and I'll keep forging ahead, making choices that are nourishing and keep lupus at bay. After all, this amazing body of mine deserves nothing but the best. And if that means occasionally having a "cheat day" where I unleash my inner sugar freak, so be it. Life is all about balance, and a little indulgence can be just what the doctor ordered.

This chapter is all about ways to find balance in the food you eat. You will learn why the 80/20 rule will help you make better food choices and when you should get help when your nutrition choices are hard. The perks of fiber will be covered, as well as why you need to be extra cautious with vitamins.

The 80/20 Rule of Eating

What makes it so hard to eat healthy? We get into trouble when we feel like our favorite foods are off-limits. Nutritionist Kristen Norton, RD, says that one reason we fall off the wagon and gobble up crappy food is because our comfort foods are taken away and we feel deprived. Combining your comfort food with healthy foods can be a great way to enjoy your favorite dishes while still eating right. But fear not—the 80/20 rule is your secret weapon here.

This rule suggests that you should **aim to eat healthy 80 percent of the time and indulge the remaining 20 percent.** The 80/20 rule is great because it prevents you from ever having to say, "UGH, I cannot eat that." Instead, you tell yourself, "I will eat healthy today so that I can have that fried chicken and waffles tomorrow."

During that 80 percent, you're eating your greens and fruits, drinking enough water, and feeling kickass. But then, the other 20 percent of the time comes around, and you see that rich, cream cheesecake topped with berries. You can't resist, and you take a bite, feeling guilty at first. But then you remember, "Hey, this is okay! I'm following the 80/20 rule, so I can indulge a little today."

For the "80 percent" part of the plan, your focus is on eating healthy foods and drinking lots of water, including:

- whole grains
- veggies and fruit
- lean protein, including plant-based proteins like beans, soy, and edamame
- avocado and olive oil fats, in moderation

Treats, or the "20 percent," should be eaten occasionally and in moderation. Take chocolate cake and wine as an example. You could have some chocolate today and a glass of wine tomorrow, but ideally not both at the same time. (I know, I know, but they are so good together!)

This way of eating is easier to maintain than stricter diets like keto diets, which strictly limit carbs and processed foods. The message is to not feel guilty about munching on your fav unhealthy foods, as you've been so good 80 percent of the time.

Progress, No Perfection

Strive for progress, not perfection, in your nutrition. No one expects you to starve yourself of the foods you love; you have to enjoy your life, and food can be a big part of this. Instead, aim for progress. Make one small change each day and count that as success. While nutrition is important, it's not the only part of your health that is under your control. There are so many more areas where your choices can have a positive impact.

Freirich suggests not relying on sheer motivation to eat healthy. Instead, set up habits and schedules in your routine so that you don't use extra energy deciding what to eat each time. What helps here is to create a weekly meal plan, have prepared frozen food saved for potential flare-ups, drink water at set times throughout your day, and keep your home stocked with food that is equally enjoyable and healthy.

Your Gut

Your digestive system plays a key role in managing your lupus disease activity. This is because 80 percent of your immune system is regulated in your stomach, small intestines, and large intestines (aka the gut). Fascinating stuff, huh? Your gut has a direct connection to your lupus and overall health. Your digestive tract is filled with over a thousand different types of bacteria, and they play a vital role in regulating the immune system. Everything you eat can have a positive or negative impact on your gut's microbiome. Like most parts of your health, the goal is to maintain a balanced population of bacteria.

Research points to the possibility that there may be a difference in the microbiome in those with lupus in comparison to healthy individuals.[53] Individuals with lupus have an abnormal mix of bacteria, and a particular type of bacteria may contribute to flare-ups.[54][55]

Fiber

Let's talk about fiber for a moment because it plays an important role in a healthy gut. Fiber is like the superhero of the digestive system, swooping in to save the day when things get a little, uh, backed up. It's like the Velcro of your colon, grabbing onto waste and sweeping it out like a boss. **Eating more foods high in fiber can also help people with SLE.**[56]

Fiber is a type of carbohydrate found only in plants, seeds, and whole grains. Lentils, avocados, chia seeds, beans, and chickpeas are some of the top fiber-rich foods. The cool thing about these foods is that they offer fiber benefits no matter if they are fresh, canned, or frozen.

A fiber-rich diet offers great health perks that include lowering cholesterol and risk factors for heart disease, controlling blood sugar, helping with weight loss, and protecting against breast cancer. A large fiber study found that eating foods high in fiber also reduced the incidence of heart disease, stroke, type 2 diabetes, and colorectal cancer by 16–24 percent.[57]

Most Americans only eat fifteen grams of fiber per day, well below the recommended 25–30 grams, which has serious health consequences beyond being constipated. Sure, dietary fiber supplements can help you reach this number, but don't rely on them for all of your fiber requirements because natural food is better. But watch out—adding fiber too quickly and/or without enough water can leave you farting, cramping, or backed up. No one wants this, so be sure to take it easy when introducing fiber and drink plenty of water.

Medication Considerations

It's important to know that some lupus medicines can make your body run out of important nutrients. These can be fixed by eating foods high in vitamins and minerals or by taking specific supplements. Find out what nutrients you might lose from each drug and work on boosting them in your diet. Here are some common lupus drugs and the vitamin deficiencies that can result from taking them.

Vitamin D deficiency is common in women with lupus, and research is still underway to see if this vitamin makes you more likely to get SLE and if your SLE symptoms worsen.[58] Vitamin D is crucial for the proper handling of calcium in the body because the body can only absorb calcium when it is present. (This explains why I am both low in this and calcium.) Low vitamin D levels make you more vulnerable to infections. Foods rich in this can be found in eggs, mushrooms, fatty fish, and fortified foods, or they can be taken in vitamin form. Your physician can guide you on how much to take based on your current levels.

Steroids, like prednisone, deplete vitamins A, B12, C, and D, folic acid, calcium, chromium, magnesium, potassium, selenium, and zinc. You may retain fluid with this drug, so keeping your meals low in salt will help with this issue. As your calcium level drops, eat foods like yogurt, milk, salmon, and broccoli to make up for this loss. Other possible side effects of prednisone include increased cholesterol and blood sugar, so it's important to keep an eye on your sugar and fat intake.

Anti-inflammatories, like NSAIDs, Celebrex, and naproxen, deplete folic acid. You can boost your intake by eating leafy vegetables like broccoli and spinach, legumes, and orange juice. For the majority, simply eating more of these foods won't be enough to make up for the folate that you've lost, and a supplement can be added.

When to Get Food Help

Anytime your nutrition begins to feel overwhelming, you should reach out for help from a registered dietitian. They are experts in food and nutrition and are trained to make food more approachable. Most major insurance companies cover the costs of seeing a registered dietitian, making this a financial and physical perk for managing lupus. Not all RDs accept all health insurance, so call ahead to confirm before visiting.

Five reasons why you might want to seek out the help of a registered dietitian:

1. Eating has become a chore or burden.
2. You're experiencing any type of digestive complaint—don't just Google it.
3. You're dealing with unhealthy thoughts or behaviors around food.
4. You have abnormal blood work or have been told to change your diet by a doctor.
5. You have food allergies, intolerances, or sensitivities—let's not guess your way through it.

Vitamins, Herbs, and Supplements

Did you know that almost two-thirds of American adults' pop dietary supplements like candy? Dietary supplements mean everything from vitamins to herbs. Recently, my neurologist told me to take a vitamin B12 supplement to help with my neuropathy. When I asked about the brand to use and the dose, his response was, "They're all the same. Just pick one." Um, no, they are not. If you've wandered down the vitamin aisle at CVS, you know there are a ton of options that all look the same. How do you know if one is better than the other? And how do you know if it's really good for your health?

What's really in those supplements, you ask?

It is a "buyer beware" situation when it comes to the supplement market, says physician Kara Wada, MD. She is a board-certified pediatric and adult allergy, immunology, and lifestyle medicine physician who learned this the hard way when she had a run-in with a superfood supplement that left her with wicked liver inflammation. Wada is not alone in this, as there's been a recent spike in liver toxicity resulting from herbal remedies and dietary supplements, which are to blame for 20 percent of all reported liver damage.[59]

My friend, don't let those supplements fool you. You can get yourself into some serious trouble with those little pills. Too high a dose can cause issues both now and over time. And don't even get me started on the toxic ingredients some of these supplements contain. They might not have the right amount of the ingredients listed on the label. And even if they do, they could still cause some major side effects. So, if you're thinking about adding more supplements to your healthy routine, remember that you're also increasing the risk of medication interactions.

When it comes to prescription medications, you can be sure that the FDA has thoroughly tested them; however, dietary supplements are a different matter. The sad truth is that the FDA doesn't have the resources to confirm if the supplements contain what they claim or if they're tainted with nasty substances like heavy metals, bacteria, or pesticides. This is where ConsumerLab.com, NSF International, and the US Pharmacopeia (USP) come in as superheroes to offer supplement advice from reputable sources that prioritize quality and safety.

Finally, when searching for supplements, don't expect your physician or pharmacist to know best. They may not be aware of the potential risks of a particular brand and could overlook potential problems like interactions with prescription medications. When in doubt, turn to an integrative or functional medicine physician for guidance.

Keep Your Doc in the Loop

Alert your rheumatologist and PCP to any changes to your diet. They don't necessarily have to approve of how you eat, but they do need to be aware of it. Ask if any problems are expected or if there is a clear reason why you should not eat a certain way for your health. And, as always, talk to your rheumatologist about adding any new supplements.

Healthy Eating Considerations: Organic awareness

By now, we all should know that organic fruits and veggies offer superb nutrition with less toxic risk, right? Brace yourself: I'm going to share something that will rock your world. Organic foods are not the be-all and end-all that they suggest. "There is a strong general consensus among nutritional science experts that eating organic foods has no considerable health benefit," says author Rina Raphael. Don't feel bad if you believed this was true. I spent an embarrassing amount of money thanks to organic food marketing.

The organic food industry is really good at using scare tactics and exploiting our emotional ties to food. Let's just say that it's so easy to get sucked in. Why wouldn't you eat spinach that had less residue and pesticides on it?

The truth is that the difference between food and poison is in the amount eaten. People need to understand that all foods, chemicals, and substances can be safe in one amount and dangerous in another. Water serves as a great example here. It's vital and necessary for life, but it can also take your life if you drink too much too quickly.

So continue to eat your organic strawberries or not—the choice is yours to make. What matters is that you still eat foods that are important for your health. If not being able to eat an organic tomato, for example, stops you from eating any of them, this is a big concern because a regular old tomato offers benefits too.

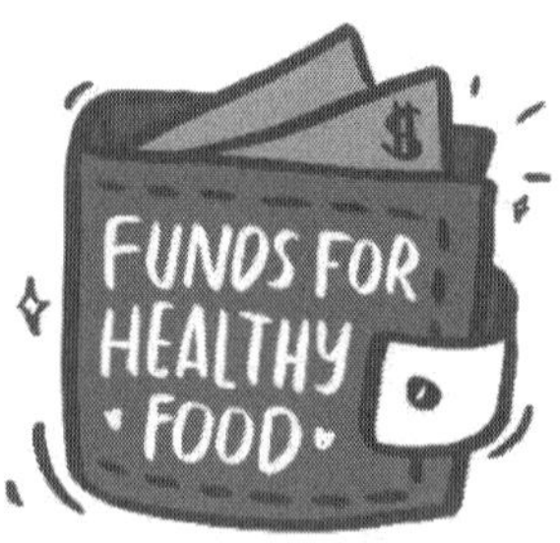

Eating healthy is expensive

Let's acknowledge the obvious: eating healthy can be expensive. It stinks that highly processed foods, which are so low in nutrients and high in calories, are also the cheapest to buy. It's no surprise that our country is dealing with an obesity crisis, given the correlation between being overweight and serious health issues like an increased risk of cancer, stroke, and heart disease, not to mention the associated high financial costs and premature death.[60]

But if you think wellness is expensive, try illness. It's damn expensive. Both forms of health come at a price. Your body (and wallet) will suffer no matter what type of food you eat.

Sure, inexpensive foods won't break the bank. But when these are your main sources of nutrition, they will undoubtedly drag you down. Then you'll pay for it in the form of poor health. Choosing foods that are packed full of nutrients and low in additives benefits you in the long run on so many levels. Fresh fruit, nuts, eggs, and olive oil are good examples of affordable foods that fit this description.

Clearly, food plays a vital role in health and fighting inflammation for women with lupus.

Reflections

- Make healthy choices 80 percent of the time and indulge the other 20 percent.
- Get help from a registered dietitian if you have trouble eating right.
- Organic food is not always better for you.
- Eating healthy is pricey, but your health is worth it in the end.

21

Let's Get Physical

Exercise gives you endorphins.
Endorphins make you happy.

—Elle Woods

I'm not claiming to be the fittest person in the world, but if you sliced me open, a dumbbell might just fall out. Growing up, I played all kinds of sports and trained like a maniac for countless 5Ks, half-marathons, and triathlons. I used to run ten miles at the crack of dawn with friends, then head to CrossFit to beat myself up even more. And yeah, I wore some stupid-ass shirts that said "No Pain, No Gain" and "Suck it Up, Buttercup."

There was a time when I could do fifty pull-ups and give my husband a piggyback around the neighborhood (don't ask me how I even thought of doing this). I did all of this and more in the pursuit of "health" and wanting to look good. Looking back, it's evident that my intensity bordered on madness.

However, autoimmune diseases forced me to slow down, or rather, my body slammed me into change. I did not give up without a fight, that's for certain. The transitions were met with kicks and spitting, but I slowly adapted.

I bid farewell to teaching the outdoor boot camps and extreme fitness classes that brought me such joy. I retired my running shoes—that one hurt. Instead, I joined yoga classes and positioned myself at the back to tame my competitive beast. And I gave myself more time to rest between workouts. My body, in turn, responded surprisingly well. While I feared transforming into a dough ball, my body held firm. Most importantly, my mind grew resilient.

This chapter will explore the incredible benefits of exercise for ladies with lupus, considering the unique needs and limitations that may arise due to the disease. While it may seem counterintuitive to engage in physical activity when faced with the challenges of this chronic autoimmune disease, research and personal experiences have shown that exercise can be a game-changer in managing SLE symptoms and improving overall well-being.

Dust Off That Leotard, Lady. We're Jumping into Fitness.

I totally know what you're thinking. UGH. Really?! Do you have to talk about exercise? That shit sucks. Before I lose you, the answer is a firm "Yep," because fitness is one of your best ways to manage SLE, lower inflammation, strengthen your brain, and improve fatigue.

Exercise is a topic that brings a visceral love or hate feeling to so many, certainly those with lupus. It's a touchy topic, as some women with lupus may just be getting by in life, yet they are expected to find the motivation and energy to exercise on top of all of the crap they deal with.

I know exercise can seem like a daunting task, but it's super important to this whole health and wellness equation. **The good news is that it's never too late to add some movement to your daily routine and get the health benefits that come with it.** Let's get moving, shall we?

Good News for Lupus

Exercise was once a big no-no for people with lupus, but now it's considered an essential part of disease management. The American College of Rheumatology says that not only is exercise safe for people with lupus, it also offers significant benefits and should be considered part of one's disease management plan.[61] Exercise reduces inflammation, makes muscles stronger, and keeps joints lubricated. Your blood flow goes up, and this helps the pain go down. It's a win-win situation for that lovely bod of yours.

Not only can you exercise with lupus, but you should!

Here's another point that is vital: Being inactive is twice as dangerous as being obese.[62] It exacerbates lupus and further lowers your overall health. People with autoimmune disorders are typically less active and more sedentary than the general public. Roughly 60 percent of those with autoimmune diseases do not reach the recommended 150 minutes of physical activity each week. It might make you feel better to know that the CDC says that only 21.7 percent of all Americans meet this goal.[63]

And there's this: If you exercise, you're less likely to die. Science shows that physical activity lowers death rates, no matter who you are or how old you are.[64]

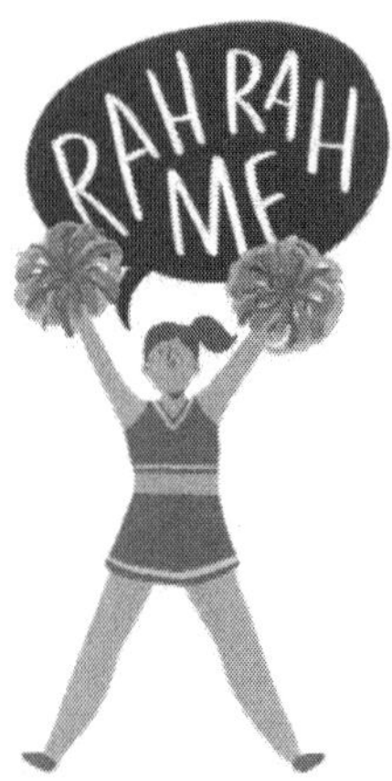

As a female with lupus, incorporating exercise into your life may require a bit more caution, but it's totally doable. Exercise can bring a lot of positive changes, from physical to emotional to social. But fear not; working out with lupus doesn't have to be that difficult—there are many workout options available that won't break your body, spirit, or wallet.

How Exercise Helps

Now I bet you are pondering: How exactly can working out be such a miracle worker for lupus? Good question. It offers a two-for-one deal for your body and mind by making your muscles more toned (hello, beach body), but it also improves blood flow, removes damaged cells, rallies those immune cells, and much more.

Physical boost

- A crucial advantage of moving your body is reduced inflammation. This unwanted bestie that tags along with lupus can make your disease worse. In a decadelong study of 4,000 middle-aged men and women, those who exercised for at least 150 minutes per week had 12 percent less inflammation than those who did not.[65] Suggesting that just 20 minutes a day is enough to get that inflammation down.
- Endorphins, the body's natural feel-good chemicals, are produced during exercise. They work by blocking the feeling of pain and are a good way to stop this cycle of pain from getting worse. Over time, this allows you to do more things you enjoy and makes the things you do every day as a part of your normal life easier.
- Joint stiffness and muscle tightness are lowered, and blood circulation improves. So, not only will your pain be less, but your body will also feel more relaxed.
- Working out helps the immune system increase blood flow, clear bacteria from the airways, and make immune cells more effective. Because of this, your immune system is able to self-regulate and improve its performance.

Brain flex

Exercise not only creates new brain cells in the hippocampus, which is responsible for memory and learning, but it also triggers the release of positive hormones that boost pleasure, alertness, and overall well-being. As your heart pumps faster, the oxygen supply to the brain increases, enhancing memory, self-control, and flexible thinking—who knew sweating could be so smart?

Additionally, exercise strengthens the brain's ability to change and adapt, which aids in learning new skills and activities, like whether or not to block your needy ex on Facebook when you are working out. By stimulating mindfulness, exercise helps you focus on the present moment, reducing mental energy spent on trivial matters. Additionally, *Joy of Movement* author Kelly McGonigal, PhD, emphasizes how regular exercise teaches your brain to handle stress more effectively, making it more resilient to life's challenges.

Exercise creates positive change and makes you stronger in the long run. But whether the stress of working out is seen as a good or bad thing depends on your view of it. If you hate working out and only do it because you feel like you have to, then it's going to feel like a total drag, no matter how good it is for you. If you think it's awesome, then it will be. Simple as that.

Flares: How Much Is Too Much?

Exercise is supposed to be a great way to de-stress, but when you've got lupus, it can be a real challenge. Your immune system is totally out of whack, and your body is under a constant barrage of inflammation, so you've got to be careful not to push yourself too hard.

The question remains: "Can exercise cause a flare-up?" And it's a tricky one to answer. Staying physically fit does, in the long run, help lower inflammation and make the immune system function better. But exercise is also a type of stress and this is a known trigger for a flare.[66]

Even though exercise is usually good for managing lupus, too much or too long of it can wipe you out and make symptoms worse, possibly causing a flare-up. Intense exercise can also cause physical and emotional stress, which may contribute to a flare. If you feel more tired, have joint pain, or have other symptoms while exercising or afterward, change your routine or take a break.

Exercise versus stress-induced flare

Some women with lupus can have a flare-up from working out. This is called an "exercise-induced lupus flare," and it is most likely to happen after a very hard workout, says Andrea Woll, personal trainer and founder of Autoimmune Strong. For these individuals, the answer is "yes" to it bringing on a flare. A flare-up could also happen after exercise if the person is already under a lot of stress. This is called a stress-induced flare. Exercise does not cause a flare-up when it is the last stressor that pushes a person over the edge.

Make changes when flaring

If and when a flare comes on, scale back the intensity and length of your exercise until your body feels better and the pain isn't growing. If you have to, stop exercising completely. You should not jump back in with both feet; instead, ease into things. After a week or two with no flare activity, you can try increasing the length of your workouts and intensity again. This is where the results are best—with gradual increases in challenges over a longer period of time. Andrea Woll reminds us that healing is a slow process and that it is important to have as few setbacks as possible.

Be Active Without Being Active

In *The Blue Zones*, Dan Buettner tells people to find ways to be active that do not require much thought. He found that people who lived a long life were full of natural movements. Activity was incorporated into daily life rather than going to the gym or doing a single workout. You can use this idea to get more exercise by parking farther away from an entrance, standing up or walking while talking on the phone, or drinking a lot of water, so you have to take many pee breaks. The goal is to make exercise so easy that there is no reason not to do it.

Reflections

- Exercise is good for you and your lupus.
- It boosts your brain, lowers inflammation, and makes pain more manageable.
- Working out too hard or too long can bring on a flare.
- Find ways to add more natural movement into your days.

22

Move That Beautiful Body

Whether you think you can or you think you can't, you're right.

—Henry Ford

I have bid farewell to the hardcore, competitive version of myself when it comes to exercising. These days, my workout routine has transformed into a balanced mix of activities, including leisurely walks, yoga and Pilates sessions, and strength training with weights. If my younger self had caught wind of this, she would have been appalled and given me some major side-eye. However, I'm no longer willing to sacrifice my health in order to look good. I may not be as physically fierce, but hey, my body loves me more now. I've finally learned to listen, take it slower, and try, for the love of all things sacred, to enjoy the ride. Deep down, I'm still a gym rat at heart, just in a more relaxed and realistic way.

Strap on your sneakers as we venture into the realm of aerobic exercises, stretching, and strength training, igniting the flames of resilience within you. Together, we'll uncover the power of activity in improving stamina, maintaining muscle tone, and defying the limitations imposed by lupus. With some guidance, you'll learn how to listen to your body even when exercise becomes too hard.

Kinds of Workouts

Assuming you're now convinced that exercise is beneficial for lupus and that it's an important piece to managing your disease, you're wondering, "Hmm, what should I do?" The three main areas to focus on are getting your heart rate up, becoming stronger, and keeping flexible. The cool thing is that the majority of exercises can offer health benefits in some way or another.

Sweat sesh

Cardio gets your heart and lungs working hard, helps you lose weight, and makes your clothes fit better. Pickleball, basketball, skiing, and even sprinting upstairs to turn off an alarm are all ways to get your heart pumping. If you're new to exercise or nursing an injury, low-impact options are gentler on your joints. These include, swimming, cycling, and using cardio machines.

Walking is my favorite low-impact exercise. You can find me walking twice a day with my sweet lab. This can be done for longer periods and is especially good for those with knee, ankle, and back issues. Did you know that walking also helps when you're stuck in a mental rut? Whatever the problem may be, a good walk can help sharpen your brain, eliminate pesky distractions, and boost your creativity by 60 percent.[67] It can also tame your sweet tooth and reduce the risk of breast cancer. So, lace up your shoes and walk away to better health.

Workout in a Group

Group exercise increases both happiness and the feeling of being connected to others. See, Jane Fonda knew what she was talking about when she created those videos. When our bodies move in unison, our minds are freed to focus on the greater good of the group rather than on our individual woes. Moving as one gives us a sense of belonging and motivates us to work and push harder. Sign up for a Zumba class or go hiking with a group of friends to double the fun.

Be All Bendy

Yoga holds a special place in my heart because it has been so healing for me throughout my diagnosis. Several weeks after teaching my first yoga class, one of the students came back to tell me that she had felt something was wrong with her body during the class. She went to the doctor and learned that her breast cancer had come back. Talk about the power of yoga!

Now, yoga won't magically cure all your lupus troubles, but it does offer up a slew of benefits. It'll make you stronger, more flexible, and happier while lowering depression and fatigue.[68] And let's not forget about the added bonus of improved posture and balance—say goodbye to awkward falls.

What's cool about yoga is that it's not just about the poses; it's like a fancy mixtape of mindfulness and meditation. You'll learn to breathe deeply like a pro and connect your body and mind. It's like finding your Zen while bending like a pretzel.

If you're a newbie, start with restorative or basic yoga. Think of it as yoga kindergarten. Restorative yoga will gently introduce you to the magic of yoga. And if you want to take it to the next level of flexibility, try yin yoga. Give tai chi or qigong a try, as they perform continuous and fluid motions, while yoga focuses on more static poses.

But hey, if yoga feels too intense, start with some gentle body stretches. It's like giving your muscles a little relaxation. Just remember, don't push it too far, unless you enjoy saying, "Oh shit!" in the middle of a stretch.

Strong as Hell

Call it what you want: resistance training, pumping iron, or lifting weights—it's a total win for the lupus body.

Strength training is like a match made in heaven for women with lupus.[69] It keeps your body safe from injuries, gives your heart a power boost, and lowers the risk of disease. Oh, and did I mention its bone-building goodness? The pressure from lifting actually makes your bones stronger, so you'll be less likely to break them.

Lifting weights revs up your metabolism for a full forty-eight hours after your workout. That means you're burning more calories even while chilling on the couch. And let's not forget the awesome perk of looking and feeling amazing as you get buff. From beach adventures with friends to some steamy fun between the sheets, everything becomes a breeze with that extra strength. Can I get an amen?

Let's address the fears and worries I've heard across my decades as a group fitness instructor. No, you won't turn into the Incredible Hulk overnight. It's physically impossible for women to bulk up like men. And those hard-earned muscles? They won't magically morph into flubber when you take a lifting break. Now you can let go of those concerns and embrace the strength within you.

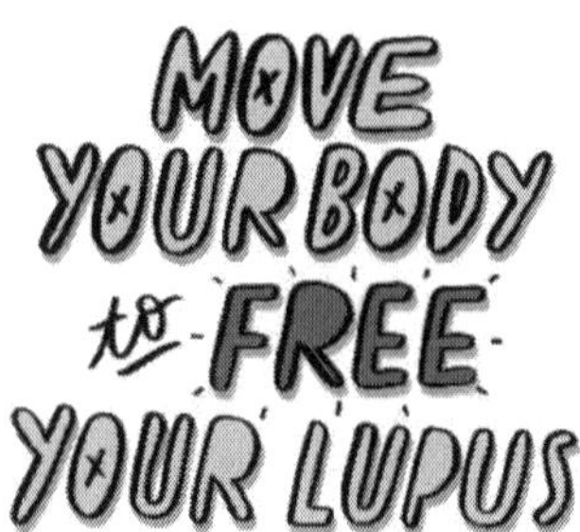

Lupus Exercise Guidelines

It can be difficult to tell you exactly how to exercise because every woman faces her own unique set of obstacles. **Many women with lupus find the best results by moving their bodies consistently most days of the week**. Pulling this off means paying close attention to your body to find the exercise sweet spot for lupus management. It's not too little or too much. It's just the right amount for you, and this takes experimentation. Start small, build consistency, and adjust as you progress.

In general, it's a good idea to follow the exercise recommendations of the World Health Organization:

- Minimum of 150 minutes of moderate-intensity aerobic exercise per week.*
- Minimum of two sessions of strength training per week that focus on all major muscle groups per session.

*Moderate-intensity is like a brisk walk, scoring around 5 or 6 on the effort scale.

If you don't have the energy to do a full workout, it's okay to do the bare minimum to get the blood pumping.

The beauty of exercise is that you can make it fit your needs. Whether you enjoy Zumba or modified push-ups, you'll still get perks. Certain exercises, like weightlifting, can offer both strength and cardio benefits with heavier weights and shorter rests.

Consistency Is Key

Here's a golden rule when it comes to reaping the rewards of exercise: consistency is key. You see, those words "daily, consistent, and regular" exercise keep popping up for a reason. The real magic happens when you make it a part of your daily routine, day in and day out.

Sure, it would be pretty sweet if a single workout or a couple of sessions could unlock a lifetime of health benefits, but alas, that's just not how it works. Our bodies crave that regular dose of movement, and this leads to long-term perks. It's the commitment to showing up for yourself, day after day, that paves the way to a healthier and happier you.

Brand Spankin' New

If you're a brand-spanking-new exerciser, even a few minutes a day can bring benefits for lupus. But it can be confusing to find the right balance without pissing off your body more. You can expect it to feel hard and challenging in the beginning. Don't worry—it's normal for the workout to feel difficult at first. Give yourself time to learn and be patient with your body.

Before going all gung-ho into a new fitness routine and splurging on Lululemon gear, consult your rheumatologist and care team. They will consider your current activity level, disease state, and overall health to guide you in finding the right approach for you. Together, you guys can determine what's right for you.

Start with small, easy exercises for short periods and aim to do them most days of the week. For example, a two-minute walk combined with some simple strength training or gentle stretches is a great starting point. Pay attention to how your body responds and gradually increase the intensity and duration of your workouts. Add more reps, extend your walking time, and make it gradually more challenging.

You may feel sore in the beginning, which can be scary if you're already familiar with pain. But remember, it's just your body adjusting to the new excitement. Keep track of your exercise and how you feel afterward to better understand your body's signals.

Trainer help

Getting the help of a professional personal trainer is a good idea if you are unsure of where to start when it comes to getting into shape. Ideally, find someone who has experience working with chronic illness and make sure they hold a national certification, like NASM or ACE. They can show you the ropes, ensure you have proper form, and guide you through the learning process. With their help, you can create a personalized exercise plan that caters to your unique body and addresses your specific needs related to lupus. Just be mindful when considering health coaches, as the industry is unregulated and lacks standardized training requirements. While they can offer motivation and support, it's best to rely on experts for precise exercise advice and guidance.

Listen to That Body!

What is most important when you exercise is to listen to your body, paying close attention to how you feel both during and afterward and assessing for any signs of excessive fatigue or injury.

Being dehydrated, having a high resting heart rate, sleeping poorly, and/or decreased motivation can negatively impact your workouts and are signs of overtraining. Learn to stop if you feel like something is wrong—not like "meh, that's hard," but "ouch, that really hurts." You need to exercise in a way that builds strength and endurance but keeps the impact on the body low. This does not often match with traditional fitness messages, and you've got to get totally fine with this.

Don't forget, even though daily exercise can seem like a chore and an added responsibility (especially during a flare-up), incorporating movement into your life can truly improve your health and well-being. Despite the challenges that may arise, make an effort to prioritize regular physical activity. Remember, any amount of exercise, no matter how short, can make a positive difference in your fitness levels and overall quality of life.

When It Feels Too Hard

When you work out too hard or for too long or don't give your body enough time to recover, this is where exercise flips from positive to negative and increases inflammation and (possibly) a flare. But it can even be more than this. If you've tried to work out and feel like, "Holy shit, this is really, really hard!" and there is considerable pain and fatigue, you may have something called exercise intolerance. Basically, this means your lupus body is less tolerant of exercise because it's already overloaded with stress and is further challenged to process it all.

It is a symptom associated with many medical conditions, particularly those that cause problems with the heart, muscle contractions, or energy levels. In women with lupus, it shows up as exhaustion, getting out of breath easily, nausea, feeling weak, and pain. Exercise intolerance also isn't the result of you effin' hating to exercise, because a lack of motivation doesn't come into play here. This isn't the same as being unfit or not having enough strength or stamina.

Being exercise intolerant doesn't mean that you should completely stop working out, as it has a very important place in your lupus healing quest. Instead, take a close look at how you are feeling when you exercise and if you are experiencing discomfort, exhaustion, and/or flare-ups. Asking yourself:

- Are these uncomfortable feelings related to the exercises?
- Do you have a flare or signs of a flare for a week or two after a lot of physical activity?
- Do you feel worse after you work out instead of better?
- After you work out, do you feel tired, angry, or irritable?

If you said "yes" to any of these, this is telling you that you need to slow down on your current fitness routine and make some changes. Learn what you can and can't do, exercise accordingly, and give yourself more time to rest. Working with a physical therapist or a skilled personal trainer can be very helpful in this situation because they can help you think of new ways to stay fit without hurting yourself.

Fit Tips for the Lovely Ladies with Lupus:

1. Research shows that **there is no one type of exercise that is better than the others**. This means you can choose how you want to work out.
2. Save money by trying out the free classes offered in your community, from yoga classes at Athleta to a local cardio boxing class. Most gyms will give you a free week to try out their facility and classes.
3. Accountability is the key to success, so if joining a gym and paying for a trainer helps you stay on track, by all means do so.

4. Use music to move your body and your mind. The most powerful songs have a strong beat, a tempo of 120 to 140 beats per minute, and lyrics that inspire. Make a workout playlist with songs like Coldplay's "Paradise" or Michael Jackson's "Beat It" to make working out easier.
5. Be kind to yourself. Some days will be harder than others; adjust your workout accordingly. Do not beat yourself up if you have to skip a day of exercise due to a flare or feeling crappy—just get back to moving as soon as you can.

Reflections

- Find ways to add some cardio, strength, and stretching into your weekly plan.
- Set a goal of 20 minutes a day to get your heart pumping.
- For the exercise newbie, consider outside help.
- Start small and expand the length and intensity as you get comfortable.

23

Protect Your Radiance: Nurturing Skin, Hair, and Shunning the Sun

If you retain nothing else, always remember the most important rule of beauty, which is: who cares?

—Tina Fey

I was on the hunt for yet another rheumatologist to take me on as a patient. My body had a lengthy trail of pain from my knees down; my fingers were so rigid it felt like I was wearing stiff leather gloves. My mind was foggy and forgetful, and I felt totally spent. But something extreme tipped the scales to make me rush to get help. I had begun to lose my hair. Hell no—not the hair!

I spent so much money on this hair, making it look all blonde-ish and such. Take away the quality and quantity of a woman's hair, and you will get one pissed-off chick. That was me. In all honesty, it was the loss of my hair that lit a fire under my ass to find a new rheumatologist, as I had an unresponsive, unremarkable rheumatologist that made it so frustrating to get the care needed.

In this chapter, we're diving into the epic battle against lupus and its arch-nemeses: your skin, the sun, and hair loss. We'll arm you with the ultimate skincare strategies to protect your precious skin from sunlight's evil powers and unveil haircare tips to keep your mane looking fabulous despite lupus's attempts to play hairdresser. Get ready to give lupus the finger and rock that SPF like a boss.

Skin

Our skin is simply amazing. It provides the first line of defense against pesky foreign invaders and helps maintain an incredibly complex microbiome. It's also the place where lupus makes its most obvious appearance, with rashes, sores, and even scarring. Between 50 and 70 percent of people with SLE have some sort of skin issue, and it can show up as:[70]

- Malar rash: the butterfly rash that typically shows up on the cheeks
- Discoid rash: red patches on the skin that can lead to scarring
- Photosensitivity: sensitivity to sunlight/UV light
- Oral ulcers: mouth and nose ulcers

Rashes

A lupus rash can take on many forms, from a butterfly rash across the nose and cheeks to a brownish rash on the body. A SLE rash can make your face look like you have a little bit of blush on, or it can appear as if you've put the entire container on your cheeks. Lupus is moody like this. For many, a rash signals a flare coming on.

You should always have a good comeback for the question, "Why is your face so red?" May I suggest: "What's wrong with your face?" or "Screw you, asshole!" Both are perfectly appropriate responses, don't you think?

Because your skin is the largest organ and provides a direct reflection of what is happening inside the body, keeping it healthy is a top priority. Overall, learn to be gentle and protective of your precious skin. Being harsh on it will only bring on more redness and irritation.

- Try breastfeeding nipple cream (yes, seriously) on extremely chapped lips.
- A makeup corrector can tone down skin discolorations. Green correctors tone down the red coloring on the face, and red ones cover the brown.
- Shower or bathe in lukewarm water, not hot water. Hot water strips the lubricating oils from the skin.

- Use an oil-based soap to boost moisture in the skin.
- Slather moisturizer on your body immediately after showering.
- Avoid using fabric softeners, as they can further irritate dry skin.

Think Before You Ink

Women often wonder if getting a tattoo could make their lupus worse. Are they safe? And should you be another lady with SLE who gets a butterfly tattoo?

Every time you get a tattoo, you run the risk of harming your skin, bringing on infections, and setting off your immune system's defenses. The larger the tattoo, the more intense the body's reaction may be. SLE medications have the risk of causing their own adverse reactions to tattoos. My friend with lupus got a medium-sized tattoo that resulted in a hospital stay with a serious staph infection. This shows the risk here is real.

In the end, it is difficult to predict how your immune system will respond. Keep in mind that some people with lupus still get tattoos without any problems, and I include myself in this group (and of course there's a butterfly tattoo involved). Get a tattoo from a licensed, reputable facility that prioritizes hygiene in the shop. Make a tattoo decision that is best for you.

Sensitive sun

It is estimated that two-thirds of people with lupus have photosensitivity. This is a sensitivity or abnormal reaction to ultraviolet radiation (UVA and UVB) from natural sunlight and artificial sources, like fluorescent lights, tanning beds, and nail salons. **UV exposure can worsen symptoms, speed SLE progression, and cause a flare.**

Photosensitivity doesn't just cause rashes. Fever, fatigue, joint pain, and other symptoms can show up as well. For some, the effects of the sun are felt immediately. This is true for me; I break out in a rash after being in direct sunlight. Other people's sun responses can take more than a week to show up. This is even more reason to keep track of what you do and how you feel every day.

At home and work

Being indoors does not mean you are fully protected from UV exposure. All fluorescent and halogen light bulbs emit some amount of this light. In your home, it is important to choose light bulbs that have the lowest possible intensity. Replace all of this lighting with LED or incandescent bulbs.

Many workplaces have fluorescent lighting. Even copy machines can emit UV rays. If working under these lights affects you, ask your employer to switch to LED or incandescent bulbs. If this cannot be done, a UV light filter may help.

Protect that skin

Because of your lupus and your photosensitive skin, sunscreen is an absolute must. On a daily basis, wear a sunscreen with SPF 30 or higher that has broad-spectrum UVA and UVB coverage. If you're wearing other makeup, put on your sunscreen first. If you have a darker skin tone, consider a tinted sunscreen. It is less likely to leave a white cast on your skin.

According to the American College of Dermatology, it takes about thirty minutes for your skin to absorb the applied sunscreen, so patiently wait before going outside. Are you really putting on enough of that sunscreen? Because most people aren't. Two full shot glasses of sunscreen are what's needed to cover your body. Wear SPF even on cloudy days because UV light can penetrate the clouds, and you can never tell what the weather will be like later on.

Increased risk

A heads up that lupus can increase your risk of developing skin cancer and this is the most common type of cancer in the US. "Oh, wonderful," you say with a sarcastic sneer. In addition to medications that suppress the immune system, certain steroids and medications that make the skin very sensitive to sunburns have shown an increase in the development of skin cancer. Luckily, this is very curable when caught early.

It's important to discuss the possibility of increased sunburn and photosensitivity with your physician before starting any new medication.

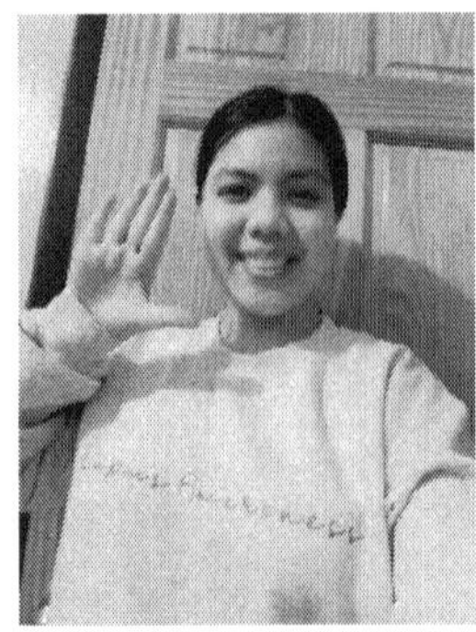

Lupus Warrior Profile

Geri Rodriguez is a New York native who epitomizes the essence of a wise lupus advocate. As the creator of @everydaylivinglupus on Instagram, she has mastered the art of connecting with her followers in a positive manner while offering unwavering support and advocacy for those living with lupus. In the realm of self-advocacy, Geri emphasizes the importance of listening to one's body and assertively seeking the necessary help, even if medical tests or physicians suggest otherwise. This advice resonated deeply with her own personal quest, particularly following a recent lymphoma diagnosis. Had she not been such a tenacious champion of her own health, the cancer may have continued to grow undetected within her body. Geri's invaluable insights extend to newly diagnosed women with SLE, encouraging them to recognize their limitations, embrace their individuality beyond lupus, and leverage the power of online support networks.

Sun tips

When venturing out, consider the following tips:

- Be like a vampire and avoid going outside between 10 a.m. and 4 p.m., when the sun is at its strongest.
- Say hell no to tanning beds—rock your paler skin. Bonus: less wrinkles too!
- Avoid the nail dryer when getting your nails done. Better yet, do them yourself and only go to a nail salon for special occasions.
- Buy sunglasses that offer UVA and UVB protection.

- Be careful because extra light reflection from snow, the ocean, or other bodies of water can expose your face and neck to more UV rays.
- Add window tint to your car to block up to 99.9 percent of the sun. An affordable option is to buy a removable window screen.

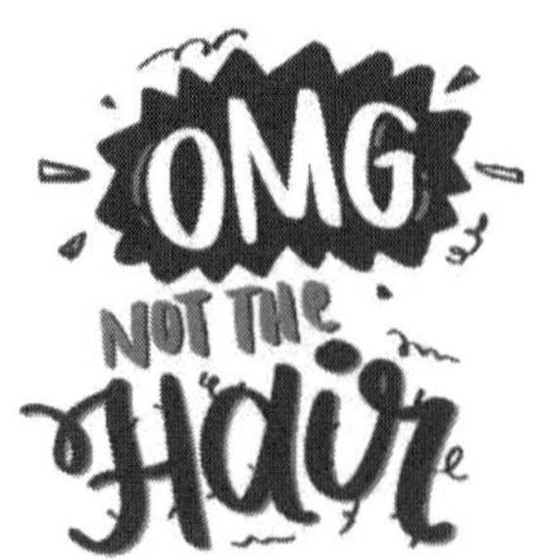

Eek, the Hair!

Hair loss is a frustrating symptom of lupus that can really take a toll. Whether it's clogging up the shower drain or filling up a garbage can, dealing with hair loss is awful. Most hair loss happens around the hairline and on the scalp, but it can also affect eyelashes, eyebrows, and body hair. The hair may also become dry, breakable, and brittle.

Statistics reveal that approximately 70 percent of individuals with SLE experience hair loss as the disease progresses.[71] This happens because the immune system targets hair cells. The amount of hair loss depends on how bad the disease is. **When the body is sick, losing hair is a way to protect itself, like skipping a period**. Luckily, when the body gets healthier, the hair usually grows back the way it did before. Phew!

Being mentally stressed about your hair falling can cause you to lose more hair. Ironic, huh? Being physically stressed can do this too. It is worth noting that some drugs used to treat lupus, like steroids, have hair loss as a side effect.

Let's pause for a moment. Losing your hair is really, really tough for women. Hair isn't just about looks. For many, hair is a sign of identity. It's the thing that you first notice about a woman, and it's a reflection of her personality. If our hair looks good, we feel really good about ourselves and are hunting for someplace to go to show off our luscious locks. When the hair has thinned out or, worse, disappeared completely, it's a downright shitty day. It's time to stay inside and watch Hulu on repeat.

Black women's hairstyles are a way for them to show who they are and how they relate to their culture. Styling hair has become a social ritual that brings people together and helps them feel closer to each other. So, the loss of hair is indeed a big fucking deal!

Hair solutions

Your hair will likely grow back. But waiting for this to happen is like waiting for your investment in Bitcoin to finally go back to its original value. And when it grows back, you look like a baby chicken for a few months as the new hairs sprout on top of your head.

Chemicals in the hair dye can act as irritants and further damage your hair follicles. Consider not dying your hair, but for me, I won't do this. I'm too vain and will gladly dye those gray hairs. If you have active discoid lesions on your scalp or are suffering from hair loss, be cautious about using hair dyes.

While there's no cure-all hair treatment here, an over-the-counter treatment is available to help grow those luxurious locks back. Minoxidil (Rogaine) is a topical ointment that must be applied twice a day to see results. Stop taking it, and you'll see your hair slide back to the way it was before.

Glamorous hair tips

Be very kind to your hair (and yourself) when you're experiencing hair loss. The goal is to keep the hair as healthy as possible.

- Use a gentle shampoo that isn't too harsh.
- Gently comb your hair or use your fingers as a way to detangle.
- Switch up your hair part to hide some hair loss.
- Forgo a hairdryer, straightener, and hot hair products.
- Tight buns or ponytails are a no-no.
- Use a leave-in hair treatment that has SPF in it.

Reflections

- Lupus can wreak havoc on your skin and hair, so be baby soft with them.

- SPF your skin all the time and stay out of the direct sun whenever possible.
- Change up your lightbulbs at work and home if you're photosensitive.
- Lupus's unfairness is on full display when it comes to hair loss.

24

Dreams and Destinations

The journey is the reward.
—Taoist proverb

Lupus, that little jerk, snuck its way into our daughter's graduation trip to Italy in July. Cramming ourselves into the tiny Fiat car, we explored the enchanting towns of Alberobello, Lecce, and Matera. We ate delicious seafood freshly plucked from the sea, marveled at the size of their huge lemons, and swam in their azure waters.

While this may sound like a dream, the reality was far from perfect. Stress levels were through the roof. Our relentless travel schedule left us exhausted as we pushed ourselves nonstop for two weeks. The scorching temperatures, soaring up to a hundred degrees, only made it worse.

Lupus wreaked havoc on my daughter's body, and every night she cried from the pain. One day, her agony reached its peak, and instead of offering the comfort she sought, my lack of empathy only made her suffering worse. In a moment of frustration, she lashed out, saying, "Mom! You, of all people, should understand what I'm going through. Why can't you be nicer?"

Ouch, that hurt. But it wasn't untrue. Not only had I lost touch with what she was going through, but I had also driven our family to exhaustion in my pursuit of experiencing everything Italy had to offer.

While I offered my promise to do better going forward, I took her words to heart. After the trip, we sat down and came up with ways to make travel easier with lupus as a sidekick, and we agreed to keep each other accountable when traveling going forward.

Welcome to the sleep sanctuary and travel survival guide for lupus warriors. In this chapter, you'll unlock the secrets to a restful night's sleep because, let's face it, beauty sleep is not just a saying. It's a superpower for managing lupus. You will learn how to give yourself ninja-level travel skills so you can plan for and handle stressful situations on your trips around the world. Get ready to slumber like a boss and conquer the world, one dream and one destination at a time.

Sleep and Health: Closely Linked

"Sleep is fundamental to life: It improves our mental being, physical health, performance, and energy," says Sahil Chopra, MD, co-founder of Empower Sleep. **Better sleep goes a long way toward making lupus more manageable,** as you're more tolerant of pain and your immune system is stronger. On the flip side, a lack of sleep is often a trigger for a flare-up.

Think of sleep as a housekeeper cleaning up your brain and body from the damage done during the day. Toxins are removed, and brain fog and fatigue can improve. "Studies have convincingly proven that sleep habits ultimately rule everything about you: how big your appetite is, how fast your metabolism runs, the strength of your immune system, how insightful you can be, and how well you cope with stress," says Sanjay Gupta, MD, in *Keep Sharp*. If you do not get enough shut-eye, you may find it difficult to concentrate and struggle with more complex mental tasks. A lack of sleep can also cause inflammation in the body, showing up as muscle aches and pains and worsening inflammatory conditions.

Sleep problems affect between 50 and 90 percent of women with chronic pain, which brings daytime fatigue, depression, and problems at work and at home.[72] Not getting enough sleep can make pain worse, creating a vicious cycle in which it keeps people awake. People often think that pain keeps them from sleeping, but the connection between the two is more complicated than that.

Women with lupus are more likely to experience sleep disturbances due to the pain of the disease. The less you sleep, the more sensitive you'll be to pain.

Don't assume that your fatigue and sleep issues are directly related to your SLE because they can result from other issues, like an out of whack thyroid or a medication side effect. Work with your physician to dig deeper and find the root causes of your sleep issues. For instance, fatigue can be both a symptom of lupus and a result of inflammation and central nervous system involvement.

Sleep disorders

Nishi Bhopal, MD, a psychiatrist and sleep physician, says that if you have an autoimmune disease, you are more likely to get sleep apnea, narcolepsy, and/or restless leg syndrome.

- Women are frequently undiagnosed with **sleep apnea**. Typical symptoms of this include difficulty falling asleep, staying asleep, or having unrefreshed sleep.
- While most people think that the hallmark symptom of **narcolepsy** is falling asleep without warning, women often present with chronic fatigue, low energy, and an inability to focus. On average, it takes 17 years to receive this diagnosis.
- Finally, **restless leg syndrome** (RLS) is more than just annoying; it's a major disruptor of sleep with no one specific cause. Sleep disorders like sleep apnea can trigger the symptoms of RLS or make them worse.

Insomnia Help

Insomnia is the most commonly diagnosed sleep disorder. At least 50 percent of people with this also suffer from chronic pain.

Cognitive behavioral therapy (CBTI-) is the first line of defense for insomnia, with as many as 50 to 60 percent of patients experiencing improvements and achieving remission in a six to twelve-month span.[73] CBT-I can be offered in a direct meeting, a group setting, online, or through an app like Sleepio, Somryst, or Dr. Lullaby. During treatment, you work with a trained clinician to identify thoughts, feelings, and behaviors that are contributing to the symptoms of insomnia. The goal of CBT-I is to help you gain long-term skills that improve your sleep as you explore the connection between the way you think, the things you do, and how you sleep.

Fundamentals of Sleep

When it comes to promoting healthy sleeping habits, Bhopal identified four key areas that go far beyond the conventional advice of maintaining a regular bedtime and include the body clock, sleep drive, nervous system, and nutrition.

Your body's clock

The part of your brain that controls your internal clock, known as the circadian rhythm cycle, is sensitive to light and darkness. Spend five to ten minutes in direct sunlight, preferably before 10 a.m., each day. This helps reset your internal clock, boosts your mood, and acts as an antidepressant. If early morning sunlight isn't doable, consider using a light therapy machine. It also helps to stick to a consistent lunchtime to keep your body's clock in sync and keep your home dark after 7 p.m. to support your body's internal clock.

Sleep drive

Sleep drive is the natural pressure to go to sleep that builds up the longer you stay awake. Wait until you feel genuinely sleepy before going to bed, regardless of the time. If you wake up early and feel anxious, watch TV or read in another room. If you're not worried, no problem—stay in your cozy bed and know that this happens to everyone every once in a while.

Nervous system

Examine your mindset around sleep and its impact on your nervous system. Be curious about your views on stress to figure out what's going on here. Avoid forcing sleep when you're not tired—the more effort you put into it, the harder it will be to actually sleep. Instead, do things that you find relaxing to keep your body chilled out.

Food and the gut

Nutrition and gut health are linked to sleep, although specifics are still being studied.

Avoid eating a lot of sugar before bedtime, as it can disrupt sleep and cause daytime sleepiness. On the other hand, fiber-rich diets help people sleep better and feel less tired.

Practice mindful eating by slowing down, savoring flavors, and chewing thoroughly. This helps calm down both the nervous system and the parasympathetic system, setting the stage for better sleep.

Sleep help and drugs

If you've followed the suggestions mentioned earlier and are still struggling with sleep, it's a good idea to visit your PCP to talk about your symptoms and undergo blood tests to rule out any underlying issues that may be affecting your sleep. If everything appears normal, you can request a referral for a sleep study. Keep in mind that you may need to advocate for yourself to get this referral, as sleep-related knowledge among healthcare professionals can be limited. Alternatively, you can explore options like Empower Sleep, a home sleep company that delivers this equipment to your doorstep.

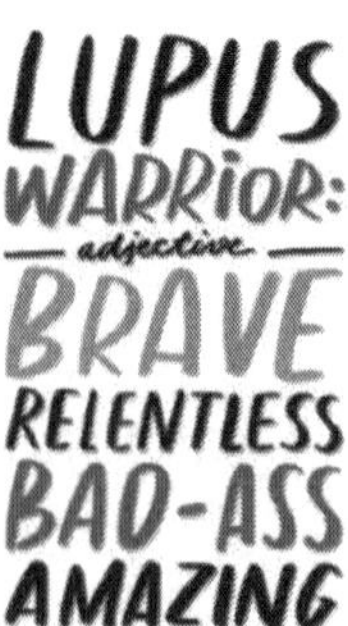

It's important to note that PCPs often address sleep issues by prescribing sleep medications such as Ambien. While these medications can be useful tools in your sleep toolkit, it's recommended to use them for a maximum of two weeks. Sleeping pills do not help you sleep much better. Most people who take sleep aids only fall asleep a few minutes faster, usually between eight and twenty minutes faster than those who do not take any medicine. Also, prescription sleep aids can have significant side effects like falling asleep or sleep eating, and they should only be used temporarily to help with sleep. Considering the associated risks, is this minimal improvement really worth it? Before starting any prescription sleep medication, collaborate with your PCP to establish a plan for discontinuing the medication within a short timeframe.

Travel On, My Friend

I have a deep love for traveling and the excitement it brings, but I have come to realize that it can also be a trigger for my flares. I often push myself too hard, wanting to experience everything and do too much, but I have learned to accept the limitations of my body and appreciate what I can do. It's disheartening, but stress is an inevitable part of travel.

I have found solace in knowing that I'm not alone in this struggle, as many other women also consider travel a trigger for their lupus. Changes in the environment can aggravate lupus activity, and the risk of illness grows with changes in diet, sleep patterns, and exposure to new bacteria. The stress of dealing with travel obstacles and unexpected cancellations can take a toll on anyone, but those with lupus are even more vulnerable. Don't worry, though. You (and I) can still enjoy traveling with proper planning.

Healthy travel tips

After that challenging trip to Italy, here are the travel tips my daughter and I created for better lupus health:

Pace yourself. When you visit a new place, it's tempting to get caught up in the excitement and try to do it all. But remember, you can't see and do everything. So, it's important to pace yourself and avoid rushing. Even if you feel fine now, pushing yourself too hard has consequences. Take your time, rest frequently, and savor the wonderful things around you—the sights, sounds, and food. My favorite way to soak up the local culture is through people-watching. Sit back with a cup of tea, check out how people dress and interact, and embrace the experience at a relaxed pace.

Dedicate a full day to rest for every two to three days of travel. This means skipping the sights and activities and instead resting up, lying low, and drinking lots of water (not margaritas). The goal is to allow yourself to recuperate and get a good night's sleep. During this down time, a massage or heat therapy (like a sauna or hot tub) would be perfect. Take advantage of what is available to you, such as the free hot springs in Arenal, Costa Rica, or a fifteen-dollar two-hour massage in Thailand.

Learn to say "nope" more. When you are traveling with others, their habits might not always mesh with your own SLE requirements. Discuss any potential challenges posed by lupus before making any plans. Then tell them you love them and thank them for supporting you on the trip.

There will be times during your trip when you need to establish limits, decline certain activities, and hope that your traveling companions understand. The limits you set are meant to help you stay healthy. Stick to them.

Travel smart. If you get sick on your trip, traveling with someone who understands your condition can make all the difference. The unpredictability of lupus means you may need some help during your trip. Whether it's a family member, friend, or loved one, this trusted source can spring into action and take over if necessary.

Travel vaccinations

Know that it is common for countries to ask foreign visitors to get vaccinated. For those with lupus, vaccinations do not commonly make the disease more active. A vaccine can contain either a live or killed virus. Vaccines are thought to be safe and effective for lupus patients when they contain killed viral components. Live vaccines should generally be avoided due to the increased risk of infection from the vaccine. Yellow fever, varicella, polio, and typhoid are a sampling of live vaccines. In many cases, killed vaccines can be given in place of live ones. If a live vaccine is required in the country visited, your physician may be able to write a note stating why you are unable to get this specific vaccine.

If you need to get vaccinated, plan ahead and spread out the shots. Ideally, get your vaccines when you're not actively in a flare and avoid all vaccine injections when lupus nephritis is present.

Before the trip tips:

- Do not travel, if possible, when you're in the middle of a flare or experiencing another illness.

- Consider travel insurance. Double check that it covers pre-existing conditions and offers the ability to cancel or postpone your trip due to getting sick. It may be harder to obtain travel insurance if you have lupus or other pre-existing medical conditions.
- Plan out the number of medications that will be needed for your trip. Bring an extra day or two of meds, just in case. Refill any necessary prescriptions well before you leave.
- Make a list of your rheumatologist's information, emergency contact information, prescription drugs, health issues, and medical allergies. Place this in your carry-on and keep a copy on your phone.
- If you are going out of the country for an extended time, ask your doctor if you should bring a Prednisone prescription just in case a flare comes on.
- Research what medical facilities are available in the area you're visiting, so you'll know where to go if you have an emergency.

On the flight tips:

Never place your medication in a checked bag because it can be delayed or lost.

- Fill up your water bottle at the airport before boarding the plane, and drink often.
- Get up often to stretch your legs, twist back and forth, and bring some blood flow to those extremities.
- Limit your alcohol while flying. Booze it up later, if you must.
- On long flights, bring compression socks to reduce swelling and help prevent blood clots.
- Assume that you won't get a great night's sleep if your flight time is long. It's okay. Plan for this.

Home away from home tips:

- Set an alarm to take your meds every day at the same time they're taken at home. Once you're outside of your normal routine, it's too easy to forget things like this. Always choose a non-smoking room.
- If you don't have a car, find a hotel close to local transit.

- Find a hotel room that meets ADA standards, if needed. That means that they have wheelchair accessible rooms with amenities like handrails in the shower and toilet.
- Bring a gel hot/cold pack and stick it in your mini-fridge. Use it at night on your sore muscles or joints.

Reflections

- Do what you can to keep your sleep healthy, and get help if needed.
- Determine if your sleep issues are really related to lupus or not.
- Traveling can be stressful, but if you plan ahead, it can also be a great time.
- The best time to get a travel vaccine is when you are not having a flare.

Conclusion
Lupus Hype Party

We can do hard things.
—Glennon Doyle

You have reached the end of the book, which means I can finally reveal the most important thing you can do to greatly improve your lupus. Drumroll, please. The answer is that there's no one health secret for lupus. Because it all matters: putting sleep first, eating healthy, managing stress, being mindful, moving that body, and prioritizing self-care and mental health. These are the essentials in your fight to manage lupus. By taking time to know what you want and need, you'll lay the groundwork for a healthier and happier you.

In this book, you've learned that lupus is not only unpredictable and incurable; it also comes with a whole host of physical and mental problems. This invisible autoimmune disease is challenging to diagnose and uses flare-ups to crash your everyday party. It's important to understand your flare triggers and create a plan to keep them at bay. If you don't have an awesome rheumatologist on your side already, be a kickass advocate who doesn't settle until she finds the right person. Always take your medications and talk to your rheumatologist before making big changes to how you eat or the supplements and medications you take.

The healthier you are, the more manageable your lupus will be. Until a cure is found for lupus, managing the disease and its symptoms is the best way to maintain a good life.

You are the sum of the daily habits you carry out, so choose small, motivating goals to set yourself up for success. Choose healthy food that nourishes your body, work on understanding and expressing your emotions, learn to see stress as a positive, and be a choosy chick when it comes to your support team. Strengthen your resilience, set boundaries to keep yourself safe, strive to be present in the moment for a bit each day, and ask for help when you run into problems.

It's time for you to rewrite your narrative. **You're not defined by your lupus—you're defined by the life you choose to live.** When you begin to focus more on how you are healing than on how lupus has screwed you over, your entire life changes for the better. Don't waste your days longing for an easier path—that only delays your progress. Instead, focus on becoming a better, stronger, smarter, and healthier version of yourself.

Finally, trust the timing of your life and trust yourself and that adaptable body of yours to get through all of this murky shit. You now have a game plan to take control of a shitty lupus diagnosis that includes:

Step 1: Admit that lupus crashed your party and give it a nod. √

Step 2: Switch gears and see lupus as your quirky sidekick instead of a dreaded foe. It's all about perspective. √√

Step 3: Develop as much awareness as you can about lupus and how it affects you. Knowledge is power, my friend. √√√

Step 4: Take charge of what you can control—kickass self-care, managing stress, making healthy choices, and more. √√√√

Grant yourself grace and compassion as you embark on this wild roller coaster ride of life with lupus.

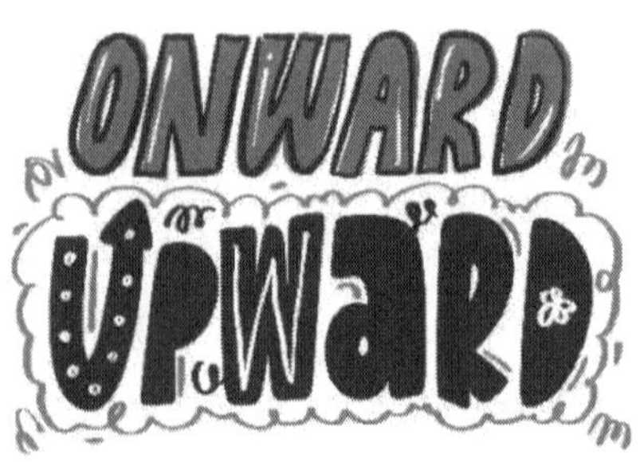

Deep Thoughts

I will leave you with a few last thoughts that will help you keep going on your lupus quest. In times of despair, may these tidbits of knowledge serve as beacons of light.

Expert you

You've lived in that kickass body for every second of your life. This makes you the ultimate expert on you. Pay attention to the subtle bodily changes and problems that arise. Be so in tune with your body that you'll know when something is out of whack. Trust yourself when you have an inkling that something is wrong—it most likely is. Don't second-guess yourself or put it off for later. Maybe you could do this if you didn't have SLE, but you don't have that freedom anymore.

Have faith in yourself, your body, and what you feel.

Agent of change

You have the power to be the agent of change in your life. Despite the ups and downs that life throws your way, remember that you are in charge. You have the ability to decide how you will act and react to whatever comes your way. Life is full of surprises and things that are out of your control, but you can choose how you deal with them. Embrace this feeling of control and face problems with resilience and determination.

Find the meaning

All that has happened to you, including lupus, has some deeply profound purpose that you may or may not be aware of just yet. Embrace the uncertainty and know that, in time, the reason will reveal itself to you. Can you learn to think of lupus as a blessing? Okay, it is not really a gift, but it is not all bad news either. Being thankful for the pain and grief it's caused lets you reflect, find value in everything you've done and what's to come, and then move forward.

Plan your life

Lupus will change things along your quest, but it can never kill your dreams. The question is: Do you really know what you want from life? Take some time to think about your short- and long-term goals for yourself, your work, and your future. What kind of life do you want to live?

What does a good life look like to you? What is on your bucket list in life? It's never too early or too late to consider these questions.

Lupus may have changed your path, but it hasn't ruined all of your plans. You just need to set a new course. Just because life didn't turn out how you imagined doesn't mean it can't still be amazing! When you know what you want in life, you're more likely to go out and get it. But if you're aimlessly wandering through life, you might settle for less than what you really want. So, if you want to run the hundred meters in the Senior Olympics or travel the world before settling down, plan it out and go for it. Lupus might require some extra considerations, but it doesn't have to stop you from achieving your dreams.

Stay open

Anything worth doing is worth trying at least once, right? Be open to whatever comes your way. When something awesome is headed straight for you, the universe will skip you over if your mind is closed and guarded. Let go of planning every detail of the unknown. Keeping an open mind helps you grow and take advantage of opportunities that come your way without planning for them. It's in these moments that you discover the beauty and richness that life has to offer. Keep your options open and your mind flexible, and good fortune will come your way.

You are enough

Let me tell you a little secret: you are more than enough, just as you are even with lupus tagging along like a barnacle. You do not have to try to be perfect or compare yourself to other people because your worth is unchanging. Accept yourself as you are, with all of your quirks, pips, and flaws. Remember that life is not a race; it is a journey of learning and growing.

It's probably worth remembering that you won't be enough for everyone. But you are enough for you. Stay in your lane, believe in your abilities, and work to be the best version of yourself.

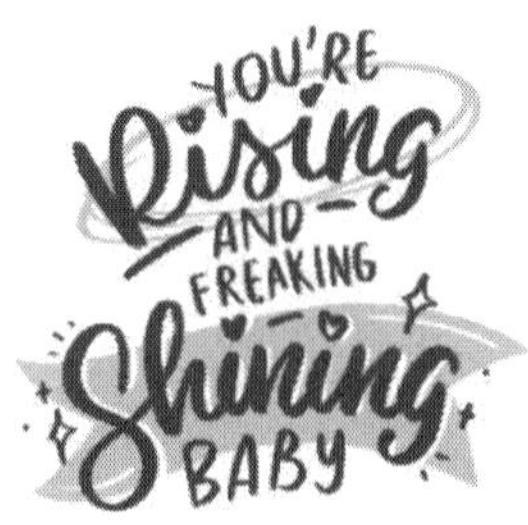

In the End

Now you know how to take control of your shitty lupus diagnosis. You have made it this far in the book, but you have only begun to scratch the surface of your potential for growth in understanding yourself and your lupus and in taking actions to improve your health.

May you always remember that you are not alone and that you have the power to get through this quest with grace, determination, and a strong spirit.

Be well, my friend. Make good choices. Forgive yourself when you don't. And remember, you are not your lupus. You are much, much more!

Gratitude and Appreciation

If there's a book that you want to read, but it hasn't been written yet, then you must write it.

—Toni Morrison

Writing this book has been the most challenging and rewarding professional endeavor I have ever undertaken. Thankfully, I came out the other end a better person for it.

When the idea for this book fell into my brain one day, I ran with it. Never once googled "how to write a book" or asked for outside help. I simply sat down and began to write—a rarity for me, as I typically overanalyze for months before beginning anything. It is for this reason that you have this book in your hands.

With a special thanks to these lovely souls who went above and beyond to help me bring this book to life: Lindsey Alexander, my editor at the Reading List, who not only schooled me on the specifics of writing a book but also was so kind when I sent her crying emails asking for date extensions. Her honesty and guidance were invaluable. Amanda Kanaan and Andrea Magee, who gave me such great marketing advice. Khanh Du Nguyen for the fun illustrations and book cover. Kimberly Campbell for her expert eye on proofreading. Kaleidoscope Fighting Lupus for their scientific wisdom. The Lupus Foundation of America for their insight, education, and support across this journey.

I would like to express my gratitude to the following people who I interviewed for the book and who also provided research support or shared their personal lupus experiences with me: Saira Sheikh, MD; Jennifer Rogers, MD; Kiran Devaraj, MD; Kara Wada, MD; Alexa Meara,

MD; Kristen Norton, RD; Tanya Freirich, RD; Racquel Dozier; Geri Rodriguez; Precious Otario; Victoria Gibbs; and Selena Colon.

My dearest Toni Winston, thank you for your unwavering support and encouragement. To my bestie, Megan Pendlum, for always being there to hear my stories and remind me that my mission is an important one.

I am so grateful to my amazing family, Noi, Kaia, and Ahnna, who tolerate my obsession with writing this book and helping women make sucky lupus better. I love you, guys!

Book Recommendations

Because reading is one of my absolute favorites, I have to provide you with a list of amazing books that have provided me with inspiration and guidance along my lupus quest.

Lupus:

The Lupus Encyclopedia, Donald Thomas (2023)

Lupus Handbook for Women, Robin Dibner and Carol Colman (1994)

The Lupus Book, Daniel J. Wallace (2009)

The First Year, Nancy Hanger (2003)

When Lupus Throws You for a Loop, Donna Oram (2017)

Overall Health

Blue Zones, Dan Buettner (2008)

The Lupus Diet Plan, Laura Rellihan (2017)

Joy of Movement, Kelly McGonigal (2022)

Atomic Habits, James Clear (2018)

Eating Well for Optimum Health, Andrew Weil, MD (2001)

Smart Sex, Emily Morse (2023)

Mental Health:

Happiness, Shawn Achor (2010)

*Unf*ck Your Brain*, Faith Harper (2017)

Death and Dying, Elisabeth Kubler-Ross (1969)

Midlife Bites, Jen Mann (2022)

*Calm the F*ck Down*, Sarah Knight (2016)

Limitless, Jim Kwik (2020)

Stress:

Upside of Stress, Kelly McGonigal (2016)

Lean In, Sheryl Sandberg (2013)

There Is No Good Card for This, Kelsey Crowe, PhD, and Emily McDowell (2017)

Boundaries:

Set Boundaries, Find Peace, Nedra Glover Tawwab (2021)

Welcome Home, Najwa Zebian (2021)

The Book of Boundaries, Melissa Urban (2021)

Breath/Mindfulness:

Breath, James Nestor (2021)

Breathe in Calm, Domonick Wegesin (2021)

The Breathing Book, Donna Farhi (1996)

The Miracle of Mindfulness, Thich Nhat Hahn (1999)

About Amanda Chay

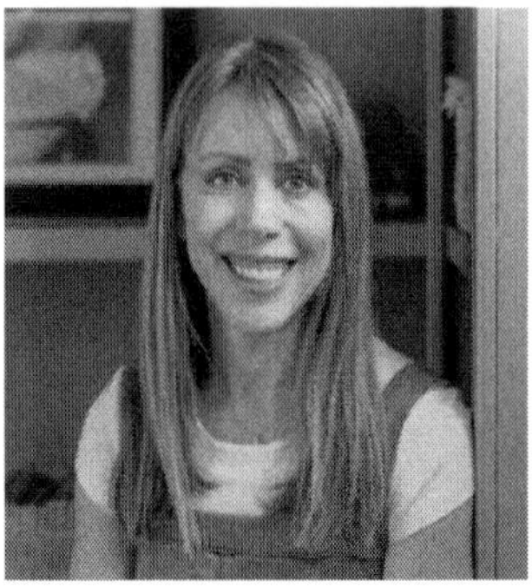

Amanda Chay is an author, entrepreneur, and lifelong health nut who has helped countless businesses and individuals put their health first. Amanda's own battle with lupus, which often drives her bonkers, has fueled her passion for helping women with lupus. With a master's degree in counseling and as the owner of a stress reduction and mindfulness training company, Amanda brings a wealth of expertise to her work. When she's not planning her next travel adventure with her daughters and husband, she's drinking jasmine tea, teaching yoga, and giving book suggestions to anyone willing to listen. Learn more at AmandaChay.com.

Book References

1. Cococaru, M., MD, PhD; Cococaru, I. M., MD, PhD; and Silosi, Isabela, MD, PhD. (2010). Mul-tiple autoimmune syndrome, Journal of Clinical Medicine. https://www.ncbi.nlm.nih.gov/pmc/articles/PMC3150011/

2. Lupus Facts and Statistics. (2019, May 5). World Lupus Day. https://worldlupusday.org/lupus-facts-and-statistics/

3. Almaani, A., Meara, A., & Rovin, B. (2017). Update on lupus nephritis. Clinical Journal of American Society of Nephrology, 12(5), 825–835. https://www.ncbi.nlm.nih.gov/pmc/articles/PMC5477208/

4. Demkova, K., Morris, D. L., & Vyse, T. J. (2022). Genetics of SLE: Does this explain susceptibility and severity across racial groups? Rheumatology, 62 (Supplement_1), i15–i21. https://doi.org/10.1093/rheumatology/keac695

5. "Women's Unseen Battle: Shining a Light on Lupus" | Health Equity Features | CDC. (n.d.). https://www.cdc.gov/healthequity/features/lupus/index.html

6. Maidhof, W. (2012, April 1). Lupus: An overview of the disease and management options. PubMed Central (PMC). https://www.ncbi.nlm.nih.gov/pmc/articles/PMC3351863/

7. Drenkard, C., & Lim, S. S. (2019). Update on lupus epidemiology: advancing health dispari-ties research through the study of minority populations. Current Opinion in Rheumatology, 31(6), 689–696. https://doi.org/10.1097/bor.0000000000000646

8. Carter, E. E., Barr, S. I., & Clarke, A. E. (2016). The Global burden of SLE: Prevalence, health disparities and socioeconomic impact. Nature Reviews Rheumatology, 12(10), 605–620. https://doi.org/10.1038/nrrheum.2016.137

9. Barr, A. C., Clowse, M. E., Maheswaranathan, M., Eder, L., Eudy, A. M., Criscione-Schreiber, L. G., Rogers, J. L., Sadun, R. E., Doss, J., & Sun, K. (2022). Association of hurried communi-cation and low patient self-efficacy with persistent nonadherence to lupus medications. Arthritis Care & Research, 75(1), 69–75. https://doi.org/10.1002/acr.25030

10. Pons-Estel, G. J., Alarcón, G. S., Scofield, L., Reinlib, L., & Cooper, G. S. (2010). Understanding the epidemiology and progression of systemic lupus erythematosus. Seminars in Arthritis and Rheumatism, 39(4), 257–268. https://doi.org/10.1016/j.semarthrit.2008.10.007

11. Thomas, D. (2014). The Lupus Encyclopedia. Johns Hopkins Press Health, 41.

12. Family and twin studies in systemic lupus erythematosus. (1997, April 1). PubMed. https://pubmed.ncbi.nlm.nih.gov/9160184/

13. Cooper, G.S., Miller, F.W., & Pandey, J.P. (1999). The role of genetic factors in autoimmune disease: implications for environmental research. Environmental Health Perspectives, 107(suppl 5), 693–700. https://doi.org/10.1289/ehp.99107s5693

14. Parks, C. G., & De Roos,A.(2014d). Pesticides, Chemical and industrial exposures in relation to systemic lupus erythematosus. Lupus, 23(6), 527–536. https://doi.org/10.1177/0961203313511680

15. Epstein-Barr Virus and Autoimmune Diseases. (2018b, May 1). National Institutes of Health (NIH). https://www.nih.gov/news-events/nih-research-matters/epstein-barr-virus-autoimmune-diseases

16. Parks, C. G., & De Roos, A.(2014e). Pesticides, chemical and industrial exposures in relation to systemic lupus erythematosus. Lupus, 23(6), 527–536. https://doi.org/10.1177/0961203313511680

17. Rheumatologist Shortage Threatens Arthritis Care. (2021, January 5). Medscape. https://www.medscape.com/viewarticle/943438

18. Ibid.

19. Sosinsky, A. Z., Rich-Edwards, J. W., Wiley, A., Wright, K., Spagnolo, P. A., & Joffe, H. (2022b). Enrollment of female participants in united states drug and device phase 1–3 clinical trials between 2016 and 2019. Contemporary Clinical Trials, 115, 106718. https://doi.org/10.1016/j.cct.2022.106718

20. Carter, E. E., Barr, S. I., & Clarke, A. E. (2016b). The global burden of SLE: prevalence, health disparities and socioeconomic impact. Nature Reviews Rheumatology, 12(10), 605–620. https://doi.org/10.1038/nrrheum.2016.137

21. Kivity, S., Agmon-Levin, N., Zandman-Goddard, G., Chapman, J., & Shoenfeld, Y. (2015). Neuropsychiatric lupus: A mosaic of clinical presentations. BMC Medicine, 13(1). https://doi.org/10.1186/s12916-015-0269-8

22. Gulinello, M., Wen, J., & Putterman, C. (2012). Neuropsychiatric symptoms in lupus. Psychi-atric Annals, 42(9), 322–328. https://doi.org/10.3928/00485713-20120906-05

23. Govoni, M., & Hanly, J. G. (2020). The management of neuropsychiatric lupus in the 21st century: Still so many unmet needs? Rheumatology, 59 (Supplement_5), v52–v62. https://doi.org/10.1093/rheumatology/keaa404

24. Kivity, S., Agmon Levin, N., Zandman-Goddard, G., Chapman, J., & Shoenfeld, Y. (2015b). Neuropsychiatric lupus: A mosaic of clinical presentations. BMC Medicine, 13(1). https://doi.org/10.1186/s12916-015-0269-8

25. Zhang, L., Fu, T., Yin, R., Zhang, Q., & Shen, B. (2017). Prevalence of depression and anxiety in systemic lupus erythematosus: A systematic review and meta-analysis. BMC Psychiatry, 17(1). https://doi.org/10.1186/s12888-017-1234-1

26. Institute for Quality and Efficiency in Health Care (IQWiG). (2020, June 18). Depression: How effective are antidepressants? InformedHealth.org, NCBI Bookshelf. https://www.ncbi.nlm.nih.gov/books/NBK361016/#:~:text=Without%20antidepressants%3A%20About%2020%20to,within%20six%20to%20eight%20weeks

27. Ibid.

28. Burns, J., Quartana, P., & Bruehl, P. (2011). Anger suppression and subsequent pain behaviors among chronic low back pain patients: Moderating effects of anger regulation style. Annals of Behavioral Medicine, 42, Issue 1, 42–54. https://academic.oup.com/abm/article/42/1/42/4565442

29. Emandfriends [@emandfriends]. (2022, March 3). "We get it! We're supposed to constantly focus on the silver linings and believe that hard, bad, impossible things make [Photograph]. Instagram. https://www.instagram.com/p/Ca8cXjWuLY1/

30. Clowse, M. E. (2007). Lupus activity in pregnancy. Rheumatic Diseases Clinics of North America, 33(2), 237–252. https://doi.org/10.1016/j.rdc.2007.01.002

31. Herbenick, D., Fu, T., Arter, J., Sanders, S. A., & Dodge, B. (2017). Women's experiences with genital touching, sexual pleasure, and orgasm: Results from a U.S. probability sample of women ages 18 to 94. Journal of Sex & Marital Therapy, 44(2), 201–212. https://doi.org/10.1080/0092623x.2017.1346530

32. Salleh, M. R. (2008, October 1). Life event, stress and illness. PubMed Central (PMC). https://www.ncbi.nlm.nih.gov/pmc/articles/PMC3341916/

33. McGonagle, D., Watad, A., Coplan, L., Lichtbroun, B., Krosser, A., Lichtbroun, M., Bragazzi, N. L., Amital, H., Afek, A., & Shoenfeld, Y. (2018). The role of stress in the mosaic of auto-immunity: An overlooked association. Autoimmunity Reviews, 17(10), 967–983. https://doi.org/10.1016/j.autrev.2018.04.005

34. Sandi, C. (2007c). Memory impairments associated with stress and aging. Neural plasticity and memory. NCBI Bookshelf. https://www.ncbi.nlm.nih.gov/books/NBK3914/

35. Leonard, B. E. (2010c). The concept of depression as a dysfunction of the immune system. Current Immunology Reviews, 6(3), 205–212. https://doi.org/10.2174/157339510791823835

36. Chen, Y., Koh, H. K., Kawachi, I., Botticelli, M., & Vander Weele, T. J. (2020). Religious service attendance and deaths related to drugs, alcohol, and suicide among US health care professionals. JAMA Psychiatry, 77(7), 737. https://doi.org/10.1001/jamapsychiatry.2020.0175

37. Engert, V., Plessow, F., Miller, R. F., Kirschbaum, C., & Singer, T. (2014). Cortisol increase in empathic stress is modulated by emotional closeness and observation modality. Psycho-neuroendocrinology, 45, 192–201. https://doi.org/10.1016/j.psyneuen.2014.04.005

38. Seery, M. D., Holman, E. A., & Silver, R. C. (2010). Whatever does not kill us: Cumulative lifetime adversity, vulnerability, and resilience. Journal of Personality and Social Psychology, 99(6), 1025–1041. https://doi.org/10.1037/a0021344

39. Keller, A. O., Litzelman, K., Wisk, L. E., Maddox, T., Cheng, E. R., Creswell, P. D., & Witt, W. P. (2012). Does the perception that stress affects health matter? The association with health and mortality. Health Psychology, 31(5), 677–684. https://doi.org/10.1037/a0026743

40. Ng, T. K. S., Fam, J., Feng, L., Cheah, I. K., Tan, C. T. Y., Nur, F., Wee, S. T., Goh, L. G., Chow, W. Z., Ho, R. C., Kua, E. H., Larbi, A., & Mahendran, R. (2020). Mindfulness improves inflammatory biomarker levels in older adults with mild cognitive impairment: A randomized controlled trial. Translational Psychiatry, 10(1). https://doi.org/10.1038/s41398-020-0696-y

41. Zeidan, F., Martucci, K. T., Kraft, R. P., Gordon, N. S., McHaffie, J. G., & Coghill, R. C. (2011). Brain mechanisms supporting the modulation of pain by mindfulness meditation. The Journal of Neuroscience, 31(14), 5540–5548. https://doi.org/10.1523/jneurosci.5791-10.2011

42. Parmentier, F. B. R., García-Toro, M., García-Campayo, J., Yañez, A., Andrés, P., & Gili, M. (2019). Mindfulness and symptoms of depression and anxiety in the general population: The mediating roles of worry, rumination, reappraisal and suppression. Frontiers in Psychology, 10. https://doi.org/10.3389/fpsyg.2019.00506

43. Hölzel, B. K., Carmody, J., Vangel, M., Congleton, C., Yerramsetti, S. M., Gard, T., & Lazar, S. W. (2011). Mindfulness practice leads to increases in regional brain gray matter density. Psychiatry Research: Neuroimaging, 191(1), 36–43. https://doi.org/10.1016/j.pscychresns.2010.08.006

44. Hamasaki, H. (2020). Effects of diaphragmatic breathing on health: A narrative review. Medicines, 7(10), 65. https://doi.org/10.3390/medicines7100065

45. Food Insight. (2020). 2018 food and health survey. Food Insight. https://foodinsight.org/2018-food-and-health-survey/

46. Knippenberg, A., Robinson, G., Wincup, C., Ciurtin, C., Jury, E. C., & Kalea, A. Z. (2022). Plant-based dietary changes may improve symptoms in patients with systemic lupus erythematosus. Lupus, 31(1), 65–76. https://doi.org/10.1177/09612033211063795

47. Barbhaiya, M., Tedeschi, S. K., Sparks, J. A., Leatherwood, C., Karlson, E. W., Willett, W. C., Lu, B., & Costenbader, K. H. (2021). Association of dietary quality with risk of incident systemic lupus erythematosus in the nurses' health study and nurses' health study II. Arthritis Care and Research, 73(9), 1250–1258. https://doi.org/10.1002/acr.24443

48. Khaw, K., Wareham, N. J., Bingham, S., Welch, A. A., Luben, R., & Day, A. N. (2008). Combined impact of health behaviours and mortality in men and women: The EPIC-Norfolk prospective population study. PLOS Medicine, 5(1), e12. https://doi.org/10.1371/journal.pmed.0050012

49. Knippenberg, A., Robinson, G., Wincup, C., Ciurtin, C., Jury, E. C., & Kalea, A. Z. (2022b). Plant-based dietary changes may improve symptoms in patients with systemic lupus erythematosus. Lupus, 31(1), 65–76. https://doi.org/10.1177/09612033211063795

50. Hewlings, S., & Kalman, D. S. (2017). Curcumin: A review of its effects on human health. Foods, 6(10), 92. https://doi.org/10.3390/foods6100092

51. Akbar, U., Yang, M., Kurian, D. S., & Mohan, C. (2017). Omega-3 fatty acids in rheumatic diseases. JCR: Journal of Clinical Rheumatology, 23(6), 330–339. https://doi.org/10.1097/rhu.0000000000000563

52. Islam, M. A., Khandker, S. S., Kotyla, P. J., & Hassan, R. (2020c). Immunomodulatory effects of diet and nutrients in systemic lupus erythematosus (SLE): A systematic review. Frontiers in Immunology, 11. https://doi.org/10.3389/fimmu.2020.01477

53. James, W., Ogunrinde, E., Wan, Z., Kamen, D. L., Oates, J. C., Gilkeson, G. S., & Jiang, W. (2022b). A distinct plasma microbiome but not gut microbiome in patients with systemic lupus erythematosus compared to healthy individuals. The Journal of Rheumatology, 49(6), 592–597. https://doi.org/10.3899/jrheum.210952

54. Xiang S, Qu Y, Qian S, et al., (2022). Association between systemic lupus erythematosus and disruption of gut microbiota: A meta-analysis. Lupus Science & Medicine. doi: 10.1136/lupus-2021-000599.

55. Azzouz DF, Chen Z, Izmirly PM, et al., (2023). Longitudinal gut microbiome analyses and blooms of pathogenic strains during lupus disease flares. Annals of the Rheumatic Diseases. doi: 10.1136/ard-2023-223929

56. Islam, M. A., Khandker, S. S., Kotyla, P. J., & Hassan, R. (2019). Immunomodulatory effects of diet and nutrients in systemic lupus erythematosus (SLE): A systematic review. Frontiers in Immunology, 11. https://doi.org/10.3389/fimmu.2020.01477

57. The Lancet. High intake of dietary fiber and whole grains associated with reduced risk of non-communicable diseases. ScienceDaily. ScienceDaily, 10 January 2019. www.sciencedaily.com/releases/2019/01/190110184737.htm

58. Hassanalilou, T., Khalili, L., Ghavamzadeh, S., Shokri, A., Payahoo, L., & Bishak, Y. K. (2018). Role of vitamin d deficiency in systemic lupus erythematosus incidence and aggravation. Auto-Immunity Highlights, 9(1). https://doi.org/10.1007/s13317-017-0101-x

59. Navarro, V., Khan, I., Björnsson, E., Seeff, L. B., Serrano, J., & Hoofnagle, J. H. (2017). Liver injury from herbal and dietary supplements. Hepatology (Baltimore, Md.), 65(1), 363. https://doi.org/10.1002/hep.28813

60. McLaren, L. (2007). Socioeconomic status and obesity. Epidemiologic Reviews, 29(1), 29–48. https://doi.org/10.1093/epirev/mxm001

61. McGonagle, D., Watad, A., Bragazzi, N. L., Lichtbroun, M., Amital, H., & Shoenfeld, Y. (2018b). Physical activity and autoimmune diseases: Get moving and manage the disease. Autoimmunity Reviews, 17(1), 53–72. https://doi.org/10.1016/j.autrev.2017.11.010

62. Versini, M., Jeandel, P., Rosenthal, E., & Shoenfeld, Y. (2014b). Obesity in autoimmune diseases: Not a passive bystander. Autoimmunity Reviews, 13(9), 981–1000. https://doi.org/10.1016/j.autrev.2014.07.001

63. FastStats. (n.d.-b). Exercise or Physical Activity. https://www.cdc.gov/nchs/fastats/exercise.htm

64. Kling, A., & Powell, K. (n.d.). 2018 Physical Activity Guidelines Advisory Committee Scientific Report. Health.gov. https://health.gov/sites/default/files/2019-09/PAG_Advisory_Committee_Report.pdf

65. Hamer, M., Sabia, S., Batty, G. D., Shipley, M. J., Tabák, A. G., Singh-Manoux, A., & Kivimaki, M. (2012). Physical activity and inflammatory markers over 10 years follow up in men and women from the Whitehall ii cohort study. Circulation, 126(8), 928. https://doi.org/10.1161/CIRCULATIONAHA.112.103879

66. Stojanovich L, Marisavljevich D. Stress as a trigger of autoimmune disease. Autoimmunity Reviews. 2008 Jan; 7(3): 209–13. doi: 10.1016/j.autrev.2007.11.007. Epub 2007 Nov 29. PMID: 18190880

67. Stanford University. (2014). Stanford study finds walking improves creativity. Stanford News. https://news.stanford.edu/2014/04/24/walking-vs-sitting-042414/

68. Woodyard, C. D. (2011). Exploring the therapeutic effects of yoga and its ability to increase quality of life. International Journal of Yoga, 4(2), 49. https://doi.org/10.4103/0973-6131.85485

69. Díaz, B. B., González, D. A., Gannar, F., Pérez, M. A., & De León, A. C. (2018b). Myokines, physical activity, insulin resistance and autoimmune diseases. Immunology Letters, 203, 1–5. https://doi.org/10.1016/j.imlet.20

70. Research on photosensitivity among people with lupus. Lupus Foundation of America. https://www.lupus.org/resources/research-on-photosensitivity-among-people-with-lupus

71. Concha, J. S. S., & Werth, V. P. (2018). Alopecias in lupus erythematosus. Lupus Science & Medicine, 5(1), e000291. https://doi.org/10.1136/lupus-2018-000291

72. Colten, H. R. (2006b). Extent and health consequences of chronic sleep loss and sleep disorders. Sleep Disorders and Sleep Deprivation - NCBI Bookshelf. https://www.ncbi.nlm.nih.gov/books/NBK19961/

73. Muench, A., Vargas, I., Grandner, M. A., Ellis, J., Posner, D., Bastien, C. H., Drummond, S. P., & Perlis, M. L. (2022b). We know CBT-I works, now what? Faculty Reviews, 11. https://doi.org/10.12703/r/11-4

Made in the USA
Middletown, DE
15 December 2023

45684122R00137